BOTULINUM TOXIN THERAPY MANUAL FOR DYSTONIA AND SPASTICITY

Edited by **Raymond L. Rosales**
and **Dirk Dressler**

Botulinum Toxin Therapy Manual for Dystonia and Spasticity
http://dx.doi.org/10.5772/61878
Edited by Raymond L. Rosales and Dirk Dressler

Contributors

Ayşe Numanoğlu Akbaş, Nikolina Semerdjieva, Nutan Sharma, Li Jiang, Zu-Lin Dou, Petr Kanovsky, Merete Bakke, Torben Dalager, Eigild Møller, Jürgen Frevert, Dirk Dressler, Beom S Jeon, Woong-Woo Lee, Roland Dominic G Jamora, Raymond Lotilla Rosales

Published by InTech

Janeza Trdine 9, 51000 Rijeka, Croatia

Publishing Process Manager Andrea Koric
Technical Editor SPi Global
Cover InTech Design team

First published December, 2016
Printed in Croatia

Additional hard copies can be obtained from orders@intechopen.com

Botulinum Toxin Therapy Manual for Dystonia and Spasticity, Edited by Raymond L. Rosales and Dirk Dressler
p. cm.
Print ISBN 978-953-51-2851-9
Online ISBN 978-953-51-2852-6

For EU product safety concerns:
IN TECH d.o.o., Prolaz Marije Krucifikse Kozulić 3, 51000 Rijeka, Croatia,
info@intechopen.com or visit our website at intechopen.com.

Meet the editors

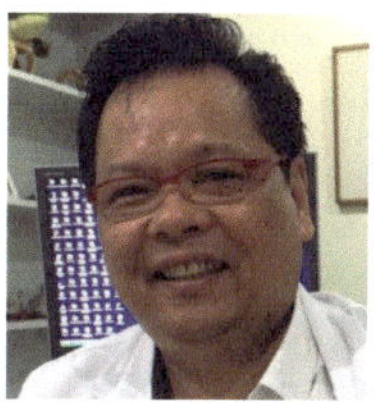

Raymond L. Rosales is a university professor and current chair of the Department of Neurology and Psychiatry of the University of Santo Tomas (UST) Hospital, Manila. He obtained his neuroscience PhD from Kagoshima University Graduate School of Medicine. He had a Neuromuscular and Movement Disorders' Subspecialty Training from the now Department of Neurology and Geriatrics of Kagoshima University (Japan) and Clinician's Programs from the EMG laboratory of Mayo Clinic and the Dystonia Clinic, Columbia University. Currently, he is the vice president of the Asian and Oceanian Myology Center and the Secretary of the International Parkinson and Movement Disorder Society (Asian and Oceanian Section). He also founded and currently heads the CNS of Metropolitan Medical Center and staff of Clinical Neurophysiology and Movement Disorder laboratories of St. Luke's Medical Center, Quezon City, Philippines.

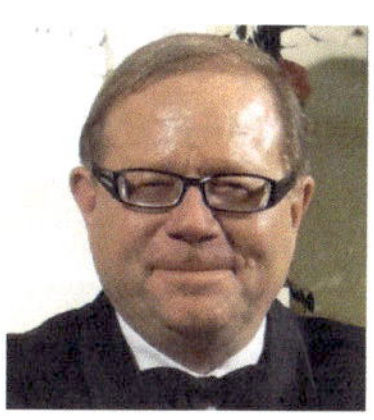

Dirk Dressler, MD, PhD, obtained his medical education at Georg-August University, Göttingen; at Friedrich-Alexander University, Erlangen; and at Harvard Medical School, Boston, MA. He is a fully board certified neurologist and psychiatrist.
He is one of the pioneers of botulinum toxin therapy in Europe. He published over 700 articles, book chapters, and abstracts as well as several books on dystonia, on other movement disorders, and on botulinum toxin therapy. He also holds several patents on botulinum toxin therapy. He serves on advisory boards of numerous medical societies and works as a consultant for various international pharmaceutical companies. He is a member of several medical societies and editor and reviewer of numerous medical journals.

Contents

Preface

How much are we ready to face our referred patients for botulinum toxin injection (BoNT) in the clinics? The challenge is there now, and it holds particularly true for cases of dystonia and spasticity alike. While envisioned to be a handbook, the clinician can handily browse through the files from a computer or from a printed book drawn out from a medical bag. Dystonia and spasticity are two muscular hyperfunctional states that could be confused from each other or comorbid in the same patient. Thus, for general neurologists, movement disorder subspecialists, and neurorehabilitation experts, this book will be a good addition to their libraries, as they face the "daily grinds" of cases with dystonia and spasticity requiring BoNT.

How can one be aided now by this handbook? The carefully chosen "hot topics" span from the contemporary basic science of BoNT to the clinical applications in dystonia and spasticity and to the skill-driven instrument-guidance injections. Be you, a novice, or an experienced clinician, practical approaches with BoNT use are endorsed ranging from "straightforward" (as in cervical dystonia and adult spasticity) to challenging clinical scenarios (as in oromandibular dystonia and cerebral palsy). Practical tips on injection planning to anatomical localization augmented by Ultrasound and Electromyography Guidance will come in handy for a clinician who could view the graphic and actual case snapshots on how to develop the skills.

Withstanding the test of time (more than 25 years) in regard to its efficacy and safety, BoNT remains to be *clinically* useful among a wide range of indications, but robust in hyperfunctional states of the muscle (as in dystonia and spasticity) and exocrine glands (as in drooling and hypersweating) and even sphincter dyssynergia (as in bladder and gastrointestinal hyperactivity). Indeed, the readers will be able to treat this book either as a primer or reference for saliency in approaching clinical scenarios. This handbook is our dedication to those of you who would like to start BoNT injections in the clinics or to those who would wish to polish your injection skills and learn how to use instrumentation guidance.

Raymond L. Rosales, MD, PhD
Department of Neurology and Psychiatry
University of Santo Tomas
Manila, Philippines

Dirk Dressler, MD, PhD
Movement Disorders Section, Department of Neurology
Hannover Medical School
Hannover, Germany

Section 1

Botulinum Toxin Therapy: Introduction

Chapter 1

Introductory Chapter: Botulinum Toxin Type A Therapy in Dystonia and Spasticity - What are Current Practical Applications?

Raymond L. Rosales and Dirk Dressler

Additional information is available at the end of the chapter

http://dx.doi.org/10.5772/66706

1. Introduction

Dystonia and Spasticity, both clinically manifesting with muscle hyperactivity, are symptomatic targets for Botulinum toxin (mainly type A, and referred to here as BoNT) injection. Certain differences exist in their phenomenology and complexity, hence the need to highlight those intricacies, as relevant in the clinics. This introductory chapter therefore aims to provide a framework upon which the practical applications of BoNT in dystonia and spasticity may be applied in contemporary times. The other chapters in this book will likewise discuss aspects of BoNT from the basic to the clinical side, including the current use of instrument-guided injections and tandem neuro-rehabilitation.

2. Dystonia Phenomenology

The contemporary definition and phenomenology of dystonia, bears the following key points, as derived from Movement Disorders Society:

(1) "Dystonia is a movement disorder characterized by sustained or intermittent muscle contractions causing abnormal, often repetitive, movements, postures, or both. Dystonic movements are typically patterned, twisting, and may be tremulous. Dystonia is often initiated or worsened by voluntary action and associated with overflow muscle activation."

(2) Phenomenology of dystonia includes influence of voluntary action, tremor occurrence, motor overflow and mirror movements.

(3) Alleviating maneuvers to reduce or abolish dystonia.

A Multi-axial diagnostic approach for dystonia includes the following:

(1) Axis I (Clinical characteristics): Age of onset, body distribution, temporal pattern and associated features.

(2) Axis II (Etiology): Nervous system pathology, inherited, acquired or idiopathic.

(3) Treatment of dystonia range from oral medications, chemodenervation (with BoNT and muscle afferent block), neurorehabilitation and functional surgery.

3. Botulinum Toxin for Dystonia

BoNT, as applied in dystonia is well established for focal, segmental and task-specific dystonias. The advantage of BoNT in dystonia is hinged on the following: (1) Dual mechanistic effects of BoNT along extrafusal (hence in muscle hyperactivity) and intrafusal (hence in posturing and muscle afferent modulatory effects along spinal and supraspinal networks) muscles; (2) Targeted therapy in focal muscular spasms; (3) Aims that improve quality of life and functioning; (4) "Tailored fit" based on the variable dystonic patterns; and (5) Repeated but robust and safe injections over time. In fact, BoNT may be considered as a "sensory trick" acting via proprioceptors, that not only alleviate muscle spasms at injected, but also contiguous areas in overflow. The usual aims of BoNT in dystonia range from relief of spasms, improve posture, pain reduction, cosmesis, and prevention of contractures, bone and joint instability, dislocation and occurrence of radiculopathy. BoNT may still have roles in generalized dystonias, where

Dystonia severity	Dystonia localisation	Primary treatment	Additional treatment	Comments
Mild	Focal	ADD/none		Inform patient about diagnosis and prognosis. ADD may be tried. If no success treatment may be postponed
	Widespread	ADD/none		
Moderate	Focal	BTT	RT (optional)	In antecollis and alternating torticollis consider DBS
	Widespread	BTT	RT (optional)	
Severe	Focal	BTT	RT ADD (optional) AD (optional)	In case of insufficient effect consider DBS
	Widespread	BTT	RT ADD (optional) AD (optional)	Either test BTT first or recommend DBS straight away
		DBS	RT BTT (optional) ADD (optional) AD (optional)	

AD, adjuvant drugs; ADD, antidystonic drugs; BTT, botulinum toxin therapy; DBS, deep brain stimulation; RT, rehabilitation therapy: physiotherapy, re-training, occupational therapy, speech therapy, sociotherapy, psychotherapy, patients groups.

Table 1. Algorithm for treatment of dystonia.

specific aims are geared to improve quality of life and functioning. An example will be BoNT for oro-mandibulo-lingual dystonias aimed at feeding and nutrition. In addition, BoNT in dystonia may still be combined with onboard oral medications and even following functional neurosurgery.

Neurological Practice Guidelines forwarded by the American Academy and European Federation indicated Level A Recommendation for BoNT in Focal dystonias, especially blepharospasm, cervical dystonia and writer's cramp. Likewise, recommendations based on dystonia severity, applying a number of management strategies, have been recently published by the IAB—Interdisciplinary Working Group for Movement Disorders Special Task Force on Interdisciplinary Treatment of Dystonia (**Table 1** from Dressler et al, Journal of Neural Transmission, 2015, with permission).

4. Spasticity and its Complexity

Spasticity may complicate stroke, multiple sclerosis (MS), cerebral palsy (CP), traumatic brain injury (TBI), spinal cord injury, hereditary spastic paraplegia a well as retroviral and other infectious spinal cord disorders.

Spasticity, as it arises from the involuntary activation of muscles, whether intermittent or continuous, may lead to pain, disability, functional impairment and eventually contractures. In the case of stroke, about a third of survivors have significant post-stroke spasticity (PSS) and among those presenting in the hospital, about half develop at least one severe contracture.

Being a complex condition, spastic paresis substantially impacts on patients' and caregivers' quality of life. Hence, spasticity management may engage interdisciplinary sub-specialties. To date, the varied rehabilitation practices in spasticity are generally aimed at prevention of secondary complications, minimizing aggravating factors, perhaps losing focus on the abnormal muscle activity itself. For instance, it is now understood that the critical factor in movement impairment in spastic paresis is the overall involvement of antagonist resistance, whether of a reflex nature or not. In addition, a wider problem area in spasticity is the fact that management should also address spasticity-related co-contraction, dystonia, associated reactions, local biomechanical changes and contracture. This present work aims to show how, incorporating BoNT injection in neurorehabilitation practices, could pave the available treatment avenues toward improving, not only muscle tone, but also other related disabilities of the paretic limb afflicted with spasticity. Majority of the discussions made hereinunder were based on our summary works on the subjects of PSS (including non-progressive brain lesions like TBI), MS and CP (suggested readings given). We also incorporated the recently published practice guidelines on the use of BoNT for adult spasticity, put forth by the American Academy of Neurology, as well as an updated systematic review of CP management (additional readings given).

5. Botulinum Toxin for Treatment Goals in Spasticity

BoNT has withstood the test of time, being an efficacious and safe symptomatic therapy for chronic spasticity, hinged from meta-analyses derived from well-conducted, randomized controlled clinical trials. Thus, BoNT, in combination with neurorehabilitation, is considered a first line treatment in focal and multifocal spasticity, both in adults and children. Pharmacologic BoNT presynaptic cholinergic blockading effects may be seen not only in extrafusal muscles, but also the intrafusal muscles, leading to a modulation of afferent signals to the spinal and supra-spinal levels. This dual blockade mechanism of action of BoNT attains clinical significance in the spasticity state where increased muscle tone and stretch reflexes occur.

Targeted use of BoNT in established spasticity should be hinged on realistic goals that will facilitate reduction of muscle tone and pain, improve passive limb functions (e.g. dressing, hygiene, cosmesis) and facilitate in tandem neurorehabilitation. Goal Attainment Scaling (GAS) may be the ideal way to assess success of BoNT injection, in that the pre-defined aims are gleaned to be person-centered, realistic and achievable. Injection protocols for BoNT should be flexible and "tailor fit" for subsequent and repeat cycle injections, considering that goals may change over time. Muscle selection with avoidance of compensatory muscles, proper dosing and dilutions, appropriate injection delivery and guidance, initial and post-injection established protocols and awareness of contraindicated disorders (e.g. neuromuscular junction disorders) should all factor in, to optimize efficacy. Improvement in active function (not so achievable to date) with established upper limb spasticity is a fair desire from both the patient and the clinician, however, one may have to incorporate the injections with an interdisciplinary team approach. In CP, patients who are malnourished and who are having oropharyngeal dysfunction, pseu-dobulbar palsy and a high Gross Motor Function Classification.

System (GMFCS) level are considered a high risk group for BoNT injection complications. In the case of MS, being an immune-mediated process, reviews state a principal suitability of BoNT for treatment of spasticity. An added benefit could be explored on how BoNT may potentially impact on the accompanying pain in MS, other than spasticity. Included in this present book are dedicated chapters on instrumentation-guided BoNT injections and rehabilitation practices in adults and children with spasticity.

6. Botulinum Toxin For Spasticity and its Associated Impairments

BoNT is a powerful treatment to address associated spasticity impairments, in that the toxin could be targeted to a muscle or muscle groups. These impairments are:

(1) Spastic co-contraction: inappropriate antagonist recruitment brought about by the volitional command on an agonist, while stretch is absent. Possibly present in usual motor movement, an excessive simultaneous co-activation of agonist and antagonist muscles in spastic paresis may occur. Muscle over-activity may predominate in some muscles in spastic paresis, causing agonist–antagonist imbalance. BoNT may potentially restore the balance around joints by focally reducing muscle over activity;

(2) Spastic dystonia: stretch-sensitive tonic muscle contraction in the absence of voluntary command to adjacent muscles and in the absence of phasic stretch of the affected muscles. As a consequence, it may alter the resting posture, while contributing to deformity and impairment of passive function. BoNT targeted to over-active muscle groups,

together with muscle lengthening, could raise stretch receptor recruitment threshold in the affected muscles and therefore reduce the severity of these potentially disabling forms of over-activity. In fact, it may well be, that this could be the best indication for BoNT injection as it addresses both phenomena of spasticity and dystonia altogether;

(3) Associated reactions: abnormal postural reactions (usually in upper limbs) seen on the hemiplegic side. These movements may posturally affect movement, as these are purposeless. Past BoNT studies targeting these undesired movements have allowed more gain in functionality amongst affected individuals, and in fact, the said improvement may become a measure of patient progression;

(4) Local biomechanical changes and contractures: musculo-skeletal mechanical changes occurring during early immobilization in an upper motor neuron syndrome that may augment resistance to passive movements, potentially increasing resting discharge of muscle spindles and eventually their stretch sensitivity. Left unattended, muscle contracture occurs by similar adaptations. In these subset of patients, muscle contracture contributes significantly to hypertonia. BoNT early injections in PSS and non-progressive brain lesions (<3 months), potentially modify the course of spasticity evolution, and perhaps prevent the disabling consequences of immobilization and contracture.

7. Optimization of bont effects in spasticity

The American Academy of Neurology gave a Grade A recommendation for BoNT in the treatment of spasticity in adults and in spasticity in CP. Together with neurorehabilitation, BoNT injections into the shorter of the two co-contracting muscles around the joint can augment stretching activities. Evidences exist on how BoNT injections indirectly modulate sensorimotor loops at the spinal and supra-spinal levels and to which end, it has the capability to modify the course and progression of spasticity, especially in early PSS interventions. The goals do change in chronic spasticity and the person-centered GAS, has been proven to optimize BoNT effects, under time-monitored endpoints.

The optimal time to best administer BoNT in either or both affected hemiparetic limbs, would be when spasticity becomes established, impeding passive and active functions, occurrence of associated reactions and pain, while impairing patient quality of life (as is true with carer burden). On the other hand, early BoNT injections potentially extend window time for motor re-learning with physiotherapy. In effect, the early BoNT intervention paradigm may potentially modify the natural progress of spasticity, prevent spasticity/dystonia-related complications or even delay re-injection.

Interestingly, a multi-modal therapeutic approach in spasticity will likely be a good model for optimizing care. Among others, those that are promising include combining BoNT injections with the following: (a) intensive occupational therapy and low-frequency repetitive transcranial magnetic stimulation; (b) constraint-induced movement therapy; and (c) high intensity ambulatory rehabilitation programs.

8. Conclusion and recommendation

Spasticity often requires consequent treatment. Therapeutic nihilism may produce devastating long-term complications. An interdisciplinary approach combines BoNT and rehabilitation. Recommendations are robust on the use of BoNT as a symptomatic therapy for PSS, non-progressive brain lesions, CP and MS. Carefully defined treatment goals are pivotal to achieve optimal outcomes and to optimize care practices. After developing the injection scheme, correct BoNT placement into the target muscles remains a major challenge. Recommended practice points to take home, when applying BoNT in spasticity, are summarized in the Table.

Recommended 10-Point Practice Guides in Botulinum toxin Injections (BoNT) for Spasticity:

(1) BoNT injections are given strong recommendations for spasticity after stroke and non-progressive brain lesions, multiple sclerosis and cerebral palsy;

(2) BoNT therapy is best indicated (based on contemporary guidelines) in chronic focal spasticity to reduce hypertonicity (and pain), improvement in disability (passive more than active functions), patient (and care-giver) quality of life and realistic person-centered goals;

(3) BoNT early interventions protocols (< 3 months from ictus) may modify spasticity progression, prevent contracture and delay re-injection;

(4) BoNT therapy may potentially restore the balance around joints by focally reducing muscle over-activity in spastic co-contraction, spastic dystonia and associated reactions;

(5) BoNT therapy should be part of a multi-modal or tandem neurorehabilitation practices to optimize achievement of goals;

(6) BoNT injections should be flexible and "tailor fit" for subsequent and repeat cycle injections, considering that goals may change;

(7) BoNT targeting, while applying appropriate and timely muscle selections, are key elements in injection success;

(8) BoNT delivery by instrumentation-guidance (e.g. ultrasound, electromyography and electrical stimulation) may further optimize injection practices;

(9) BoNT correct dosing and appropriate dilutions are important guides during injections (e.g. "high potency, low dilutions" to localize/maximize desired effects in small forearm and hand and foot muscles; "low potency, high dilutions" intended to spread the toxin in large arm, thigh and leg muscles);

(10) BoNT caveats in injection include: over-enthused injections in spasticity-protective muscles (e.g. postural thigh muscles), compensatory muscles, concomitant neuromuscular junction disorders, frail and malnourished children or those with high Gross Motor Function Classification System.

---

http://dx.doi.org/10.5772/66706

Author details

Raymond L. Rosales[1]* and Dirk Dressler[2]

*Address all correspondence to: rlrosalesmd88@gmail.com

1 Department of Neurology and Psychiatry, University of Santo Tomas, Manila, Philippines

2 Movement Disorders Section, Department of Neurology, Hannover Medical School, Hannover, Germany

Suggested readings

[1] D. Dressler, E. Altenmueller, R. Bhidayasiri, S. Boholega, ,P. Chana, T.M. Chung, S. Frucht, P.J. Garcia-Ruiz, A. Kaeli, R. Kaji, P. Kanovsky, R. Laskawi, F. Micheli, O. Orlova, M. Relja, R.L. Rosales, J. Slawek, S. Timerbaeva, T.T. Warner, F.A. Saberi: Strategies for treatment of dystonia. Journal of Neural Transmission. DOI: 10.1007/s00702-015-1453-x

[2] D. Dressler, R. Bhidayasiri, S. Bohlega, A. Chahidi, T.M. Chung, M. Ebke, J. Jacinto, R. Kaji, S. Kocer, P. Kanovsky, F. Micheli, O. Orlova, S. Paus, Z. Pirtosek, M. Relja, R.L. Rosales, J.A. Sagastegui-Rodrıguez, P.W. Schoenle, G.A. Shahidi, S. Timerbaeva, U. Walter, F.A. Saberi: Botulinum toxin therapy for treatment of spasticity in multiple sclerosis: review and recommendations of the IAB-Interdisciplinary Working Group for Movement Disorders task force. Journal of Neurology, October 2016, DOI: 10.1007/s00415-016-8304-z

[3] K. Fheodoroff, J. Jacinto, A. Geurts, F. Molteni, J.H. Franco, T. Santiago, R.L. Rosales, J.M. Gracies: How Can We Improve Current Practice in Spastic Paresis? European Neurological Reviews, 2016;11:ePub ahead of print.

[4] M.A.L.P Gozum and R.L. Rosales: Botulinum Toxin A therapy in Early Post-Stroke Spasticity: Providing a wider treatment avenue. Internaional Journal of NeuroRehabilitation 3(3), 2016 http://dx.doi.org/10.4172/2376-0281.1000207

[5] M. Lukban, R.L. Rosales, D. Dressler: Effectiveness of Botulinum Toxin A for Upper and Lower Limb Spasticity in Children with Cerebral Palsy: A Summary of Evidence. Journal of Neural Transmission 116: 319-331, 2009.

[6] P. Kanovsky, K. Bhatia, R.L. Rosales (editors): Dystonia and dystonic syndromes; Springer, GmbH, Germany (2015) ISBN 978-3-7091-1515-2 ISBN 978-3-7091-1516-9 (eBook) DOI: 10.1007/978-3-7091-1516-9

[7] R.L. Rosales (Chapter-8): Dystonia, Spasticity and Botulinum Toxin Therapy: Rationale, Evidences and Clinical Context; In: R.L. Rosales (Editor). Dystonia: The Many Facets. (Intech Open Access Publishers, Croatia), 2012, ISBN: 978-953-307-1116-8 (www.intechopen.com) (pp. 83-98).

[8] R.L. Rosales and A. Chua-Yap: Evidence-based systematic review on the efficacy and safety of botulinum toxin therapy in post-stroke spasticity. Journal of Neural Transmission 115 (4): 617-623, 2008.

[9] R.L. Rosales, D. Dressler: On muscle spindles, dystonia and botulinum toxin. European Journal of Neurology 17 (Suppl. 1): 71–80, 2010.

[10] R.L. Rosales, F. Efendy, E.S. Teleg, M.M.D. Delos Santos, M.C.E. Rosales, M. Ostrea , M.J. Tanglao, A.R. Ng: Botulinum toxin as early intervention for spasticity after stroke or non-progressive brain lesion: A meta-analysis. Journal of the Neurological Sciences 371: 6–14, 2016 http://dx.doi.org/10.1016/j.jns.2016.10.005

[11] R.L. Rosales, P. Kanovsky, H.H. Fernandez: What's the "catch" in upper-limb post-stroke spasticity: Expanding the role of botulinum toxin applications, Parkinsonism and Related Disorders 17: S3-10, 2011 (doi:10.1016/j.parkreldis.2011.06.019).

Additional references

[1] D.M. Simpson, M. Hallett, E.J. Ashman, C.L. Comella, M.W. Green, et al., Practice guideline update summary: botulinum neurotoxin for the treatment of blepharospasm,cervical dystonia, adult spasticity, and headache; Report of the Guideline Development Subcommittee of the American Academy of Neurology, Neurology 86 (2016) 1–9, http://dx.doi.org/10.1212/WNL.0000000000002560

[2] I. Novak, S. Mcintyre, C. Morgan, L. Campbell, L. Dark, N. Morton, E. Stumbles, S. Wilson, S. Goldsmith: A systematic review of interventions for children with cerebral palsy: state of the evidence, Developmental Medicine & Child Neurology 55: 885–910, 2013.

Section 2

Botulinum Toxin Therapy: Basic Science

Chapter 2

How Much Evidence do we have on the Central Effects of Botulinum Toxin in Spasticity and Dystonia?

Tomáš Veverka, Martin Nevrlý, Pavel Otruba,
Petr Hluštík and Petr Kaňovský

Additional information is available at the end of the chapter

http://dx.doi.org/10.5772/64763

Abstract

The brain is continually reorganizing (plasticity). Plastic changes within the sensorimotor system are not only beneficial (adaptive plasticity) but may even worsen function (maladaptive plasticity). Conditions such as dystonia and poststroke spasticity (PSS) that interfere with motor performance could be attributed to maladaptive plasticity. Botulinum toxin (BoNT) has been proven to be safe and effective in treating various hyperfunctional cholinergic states. Beside the well-known neuromuscular junction site of action, BoNT also exerts effects through supraspinal mechanisms and can even affect cortical reorganization. The hypothesis of central reorganization following BoNT treatment has been supported by studies using neurophysiological and imaging methods in patients with focal dystonia and PSS. The growing evidence of BoNT-related central (remote) effects make BoNT injections a promising tool to favorably affect maladaptive changes even at the cortical level.

Keywords: stroke, dystonia, spasticity, botulinum toxin, functional magnetic resonance imaging, neuronal plasticity

1. Introduction

Botulinum toxin (BoNT) type A is a valuable therapeutic option for the management of poststroke spasticity (PSS) [1–3] and focal dystonia [4]. BoNT acts at the neuromuscular junction, and the mechanism of action on muscle spindles has been well described [5, 6]. In the periphery, BoNT affects intrafusal fibers as well as extrafusal ones and thus alters pathological sensory inputs to the central nervous system (CNS) by blocking of the neuromuscular junction of the gamma motor neurons [6]. This blockade leads to a reduction of Ia afferent signals and indirectly inhibits pre-existing feedback-driven execution mode. This is probably the mechanism by which BoNT injected in the periphery may induce dynamic changes at several hierarchical levels of the sensorimotor system, presumably including cerebral cortex [7]. The hypothesis of central reorganization following BoNT treatment has been supported by studies using neurophysiological and imaging methods in patients with focal dystonia and PSS.

2. Spasticity

Stroke is a leading cause of disability in Western countries [8]. Ischemic lesions of descending tracts result in upper motor neuron syndrome (UMNS) comprising both negative signs (weakness and loss of dexterity) and positive signs (especially spasticity) [9]. Up to two thirds of stroke survivors experience impaired function and spasticity of the upper limb, and wrist and finger impairments usually prevail over involvement of proximal shoulder muscles [10, 11]. The degree of muscle weakness is crucial in determining the movement deficit following stroke, but spasticity may also be contributory [12, 13]. It is generally recognized that PSS may interfere with voluntary movement [14]. Disabling PSS affects patient's quality of life and frequently causes significant reductions in manual dexterity, mobility, walking/falling, and performance of activities of daily living (ADL) [15]. Disabilities associated with PSS place a significant burden on stroke survivors and subsequently on caregivers [16]. Prevalence data for PSS are limited by a lack of population-based studies; however, current estimates range from 19 to 42.6% [15, 17]. Numerous clinical trials have shown that BoNT is a safe and effective therapeutic tool to relieve upper limb PSS and improve function of the affected limb [1, 18, 19]. Recommended treatment strategies to relieve PSS combine physiotherapy procedures with BoNT application [1–3]. Although BoNT acts primarily on muscle spindles [5, 6], there is growing evidence that BoNT also exerts effects through supraspinal mechanisms and can even affect cortical reorganization [7]. The hypothesis of central reorganization following BoNT treatment has been supported mostly by studies using neurophysiological [20–23] and imaging [24–26] methods in patients with focal dystonia. Most of published functional magnetic resonance imaging (fMRI) studies in chronic stroke patients have described changes in task-related cortical activity following physiotherapy treatment [27, 28]. In the last decade, several studies reported central (remote) effects of BoNT in PSS.

Two pilot studies using blood oxygenation level dependent (BOLD) functional magnetic resonance imaging (fMRI) to register and localize BoNT-related changes of cerebral cortex activation were conducted. Both studies showed that effective treatment of spasticity led to a reduction of abnormal extensive bilateral activation of cortical and subcortical areas during actively performed or imagery of finger movement. The between-session contrasts designed to display the specific BoNT effect revealed a significant change in the local BOLD signal magnitude not only in traditional motor areas but also in areas that have been considered to be a part of a "broader" motor system or have only rarely been reported in the context of volitional motor control (posterior cingulate, DLPFC, Broca's area). Finally, the above-mentioned studies confirmed that fMRI is a suitable tool in studying cortical relief of spasticity and that the three-session study design permits decomposition of BoNT effect from compounding effects of rehabilitation and time [29, 30]. Nevertheless, the promising results have been limited by the small number of subjects.

Manganotti et al. [31], in another fMRI study involving patients with PSS treated with BoNT alone, reported a similar effect representing a trend toward normalization of movement-induced brain activation. Detected pretreatment overactivation in the bilateral sensorimotor cortex (SM1, supplementary motor area (SMA)) and cerebellum was followed by decrease in extent of sensorimotor activation with increase in laterality after BoNT application.

In a subsequent fMRI study based on the pilot results [29, 30], using the combination of rehabilitation and BoNT for completely plegic patients with PSS, the alleviation of spasticity following BoNT treatment was associated with reduction of the brain activation volume in response to a motor imagery. The BOLD signal at week 11, when peripheral effect of BoNT was expected to wane (BoNT-off), revealed further volume reduction (**Figure 1**). The authors hypothesized that BoNT application modifies the process of cerebral plasticity and that this impact might persist despite temporary effect of BoNT on muscle fibers. A notable exception to this trend would be in regard to the cerebellar hemispheres, which either appear similarly active across the three imaging sessions (ipsilesional) or manifest transient activation at the time of maximal BoNT effect (contralesional) [32].

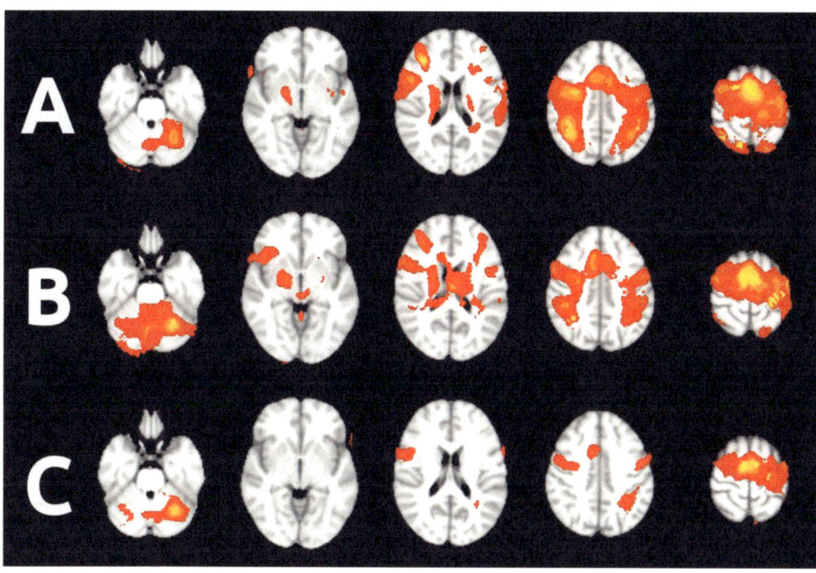

Figure 1. Functional MRI activation during imagery of finger movement (A) before BoNT treatment, (B) 4 and (C) 11 weeks after BoNT application (group mean statistical maps overlaid in color on the MNI anatomical template). Adapted with permission from Veverka et al. [32].

The following study of two age-matched groups with moderate and severe hand weakness demonstrated different effects of BoNT-induced improvement in spasticity on sensorimotor networks. The plegic group performing movement imagery in MR scanner manifested BoNT-induced reduction of activation in structures associated with visual imagery. Regarding the occipitoparietal changes, the BoNT treatment in plegic subjects might switch their neural processing from visual to kinesthetic imagery pattern. In the paretic group, performing sequential finger movement, overall brain activation was markedly reduced after BoNT. Between-session contrasts yielded significant BoNT-related changes in the ipsilesional DLPFC and Broca's area, similarly as in the study of Tomášová et al. [30]. Both areas have been reported to participate in motor learning, rather than volitional motor performance and control [33]. Several areas with decreased task-related BOLD response after BoNT-induced spasticity relief subsequently increased their activation again as BoNT effect waned. These included the ipsilesional lateral occipital cortex, ipsilesional cortex bordering the intraparietal sulcus, and contralesional cerebellum. Activation reductions over the whole three-month study period were located in bilateral occipital cortex, which may reflect the decreased need to engage visualization in order to perform the movement with the paretic hand.

Another study using a combination of BoNT and rehabilitation in a subgroup of post-stroke spasticity with residual motor activity reported BOLD activity increases in the ipsilesional primary sensorimotor cortex and in the contralesional secondary somatosensory area 14 weeks following BoNT application enhanced by three months of repetitive arm cycling. The authors concluded that observed cortical changes reflect a treatment-induced effect [34].

In a recent study, Bergfeldt et al. [35] reported an increase in brain activation in response to an active motor task in the motor and premotor cortex (predominantly contralesional) at the baseline and an overall decrease in activation with contralesional predominance following comprehensive focal spasticity therapy.

A more recent study [36] engaging severely affected patients with PSS revealed BoNT-related patterns of cerebral cortex activation during passive hand movement. The whole-brain fMRI data were acquired during paced repetitive passive movements of the plegic hand (flexion/extension at the wrist) alternating with rest. Passive movement induces sensorimotor cortex activation in another way, with particular emphasis on afferent inputs to the CNS [37]. Across all the sessions, fMRI activation of the ipsilesional sensorimotor cortex (M1, S1, and SMA) dominated, with notable temporal reduction of activation throughout the study (paired contrast pre-BoNT > BoNT-off). At week 4, when maximal pharmacological effect of BoNT is expected, additional clusters transiently emerged bilaterally in the cerebellum, in the contralesional sensorimotor cortex, and in the contralesional occipital cortex. Paired contrasts demonstrated significant differences post-BoNT > pre-BoNT (bilateral cerebellum and contralesional occipital cortex) and post-BoNT > BoNT-off (ipsilesional cerebellum and SMA) [36].

Stroke triggers a number of processes at various levels of the motor system that can cause spontaneous recovery or motor improvement (adaptive plasticity). Plastic changes within the sensorimotor system are not only beneficial but may even worsen residual function. From this point of view, appearance of poststroke upper limb spasticity that interferes with motor performance could be attributed to so-called maladaptive plasticity. The BoNT injection is a well-established component of multimodal treatment of PSS. The growing evidence of BoNT-related central (remote) effects makes BoNT a promising tool to favorably affect maladaptive changes even at the cortical level.

3. Dystonia

BoNT types A and B have been proven to be safe and effective in treating various hyperfunctional cholinergic states [38, 39]. BoNT is more effective in blocking active neuromuscular junctions [40]. BoNT disrupts neurotransmission by cleavage of presynaptic vesicle fusion proteins; SNAP-25 for BoNT type A and synaptobrevin for BoNT type B [5]. BoNT is currently considered to be one of the most effective therapeutic options in the management of focal dystonias [4]. The clinical effect of BoNT on dystonia is assumed to be mediated by dynamic changes at multiple levels of the sensorimotor system, from the neuromuscular junction up to the cerebral cortex, as documented by previous behavioral and electrophysiological studies [21, 41]. Some fMRI studies showed significant treatment-related changes in the sensorimotor network in patients with cervical dystonia receiving long-term treatment with BoNT [25, 26]. It is important to stress here that the BoNT experience from the past 20 years brought us nearer to our understanding of the underpinnings of current dystonia pathophysiological concepts. Undoubtedly, the introduction of the first-generation BoNT products (Botox, Allergan Pharmaceuticals, Irvine, CA, USA; Dysport, Ipsen Pharmaceutical, Paris, France) not only led to the breakthrough in dystonia treatment but also the breakthrough in dystonia research. We now know that the dystonic hyperactive and cholinergically sensitive extrafusal, and in parallel, the intrafusal muscle fibers are the prime targets of BoNT therapy [6]. It is in the latter effect of BoNT in muscle spindles that would eventually modify proprioceptive spindle afferents, as these are partly dependent on the intrafusal muscle fiber tensions. A modification of the central programs with BoNT may eventually occur at the spinal and supraspinal levels [6]. Soon, specialists in movement disorders clinics realized that dystonia may behave differently during the course of BoNT treatment. The first reports described the changes of the muscular pattern [42–46] that may have implied a central mechanism of dystonia. Studies that employed the long-latency reflexes and the central SEP components provided support to such central mechanisms in dystonia [21], and this would include TMS [22]. Interestingly, the cortical abnormality in dystonia (either the excitability or intracortical inhibition) changed (i.e., "normalized") following an efficacious treatment with BoNT. The implication was that a peripheral blockade of effectors may have engaged the central motor programs in dystonia. As we await more data on the probable "direct" retrograde effects of BoNT, the "indirect" effects remain tenable to date, the latter being hinged upon the normalization of abnormal muscle-spindle functioning in dystonia [6]. The consequent and apparent normalization of the cortical disorder following BoNT injections in dystonia may indicate that the manipulation of proprioceptive afferent input has a substantial impact on the disorder directly at the central level [21, 22]. It can be assumed that the abnormalities of Bereitschaft potentials, contingent negative variation, and electroencephalogram desynchronization point (with a high level of probability) to a disorder in the process of motor programming in dystonia and that these occur at the cortical level. What follows is a defective motor performance, as reflected in abnormalities of reciprocal inhibition, long-latency reflex, cortical excitability, and intracortical inhibition. Taken together, it would seem that an abnormal sensorimotor integration exists in dystonia, and this phenomenon has been alluded to in a number of published works [6, 47, 48]. The sensorimotor integration in the physiological perspective involves all parts of the motor and sensory system, including the motor circuits, in which the basal ganglia and the premotor and motor cortex are the principal components. Recently, it has been hypothesized that sensorimotor integration is, in fact, a function of brain plasticity. Indeed, transcranial stimulation studies have supported the likely occurrence of disordered plasticity in dystonia [49, 50].

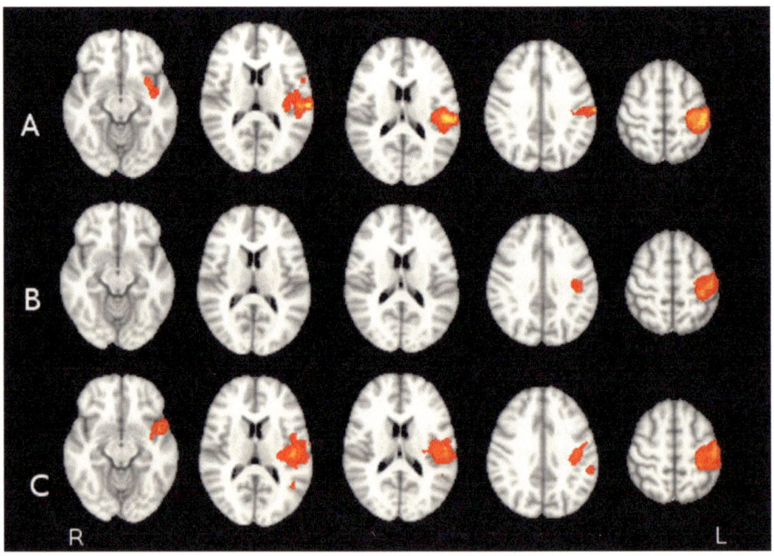

Figure 2. Functional MRI activation during finger movement and simultaneous median nerve stimulation: controls (A), torticollis patients before BoNT treatment (B), and torticollis patients 4 weeks after BoNT treatment (C); group mean statistical maps overlaid in color on MNI anatomical template. Adapted with permission from Opavský et al. [25].

Perhaps to date, the most appropriate tool to investigate brain plasticity would be functional magnetic resonance imaging (fMRI). We have seen the changes that are typical for altered brain plasticity in torticollis patients (when compared with healthy individuals) and their normalization following successful treatment with BoNT. Significant reduction of task-related activation within the ipsilateral supplementary motor area (SMA) and dorsal premotor cortex was observed following successful BoNT treatment. There was also a trend in SMA activation in patients to change lateralization from predominantly ipsilateral to contralateral after BoNT. BoNT treatment was associated with a significant reduction in finger movement-induced fMRI activation (during simultaneous median nerve stimulation) of several brain areas (**Figure 2**), especially in SMA, cingulum, contralateral thalamus, secondary somatosensory cortex, and also in the central part of cerebellum, close to the vermis [25, 26]. These results support previous observations that the BoNT effect has a correlate at the central nervous system level. It is our

http://dx.doi.org/10.5772/64763

belief that further studies will show us that the sensorimotor integration or brain plasticity represents the process of motor preparation itself, even in the expert motor performances.

Acknowledgements

This study was supported by the grants of the Agency for Healthcare Research of Ministry of Health of the Czech Republic (AZV MZ ČR) 15-31921A and 16-30210A. This work was also supported by the Institutional support of the Research Organisation – Ministry of Health, Czech Republic, RVO – FNOL 2016.

Author details

Tomáš Veverka, Martin Nevrlý, Pavel Otruba, Petr Hluštík and Petr Kaňovský*

*Address all correspondence to: petr.kanovsky@fnol.cz

Department of Neurology, Faculty of Medicine and Dentistry, University Hospital, Olomouc, Czech Republic

References

[1] Wissel J, Ward AB, Erztgaard P, Bensmail D, Hecht MJ, Lejeune TM, et al. European consensus table on the use of botulinum toxin type A in adult spasticity. J Rehabil Med. 2009;41(1):13–25.

[2] Hesse S, Werner C. Poststroke motor dysfunction and spasticity: novel pharmacological and physical treatment strategies. CNS Drugs. 2003;17(15):1093–107.

[3] Ward AB, Aguilar M, De Beyl Z, Gedin S, Kaňovský P, Molteni F, et al. Use of botulinum toxin type A in management of adult spasticity—a European consensus statement. J Rehab Med. 2003;35(2):98–9.

[4] Jankovic J. Treatment of cervical dystonia with botulinum toxin. Mov Disord. 2004;19(Suppl 8):S109–115.

[5] Dressler D, Saberi FA, Barbosa ER. Botulinum toxin: mechanisms of action. Arq Neuropsiquiatr. 2005;63(1):180–5.

[6] Rosales RL, Dressler D. On muscle spindles, dystonia and botulinum toxin. Eur J Neurol. 2010;17(Suppl 1):71–80.

[7] Currà A, Trompetto C, Abbruzzese G, Berardelli A. Central effects of botulinum toxin type A: evidence and supposition. Mov Disord. 2004;19(Suppl 8):S60–64.

[8] Mathers CD, Loncar D. Projections of global mortality and burden of disease from 2002 to 2030. PLoS Med. 2006;3(11):e442.

[9] Sheean G. The pathophysiology of spasticity. Eur J Neurol. 2002;9(Suppl 1):3–9; discussion 53–61.

[10] Colebatch JG, Gandevia SC. The distribution of muscular weakness in upper motor neuron lesions affecting the arm. Brain. 1989;112(Pt 3):749–63.

[11] Jørgensen HS, Nakayama H, Raaschou HO, Vive-Larsen J, Støier M, Olsen TS. Outcome and time course of recovery in stroke. Part I: outcome. The Copenhagen Stroke Study. Arch Phys Med Rehabil. 1995;76(5):399–405.

[12] Ada L, O'Dwyer N, O'Neill E. Relation between spasticity, weakness and contracture of the elbow flexors and upper limb activity after stroke: an observational study. Disabil Rehabil. 2006;28(13–14):891–7.

[13] Kamper DG, Fischer HC, Cruz EG, Rymer WZ. Weakness is the primary contributor to finger impairment in chronic stroke. Arch Phys Med Rehabil. 2006;87(9):1262–9.

[14] Mayer NH, Esquenazi A, Childers MK. Common patterns of clinical motor dysfunction. Muscle Nerve Suppl. 1997;6:S21–35.

[15] Sommerfeld DK, Eek EU-B, Svensson A-K, Holmqvist LW, Von Arbin MH. Spasticity after stroke: its occurrence and association with motor impairments and activity limitations. Stroke. 2004;35(1):134–9.

[16] Zorowitz RD, Gillard PJ, Brainin M. Poststroke spasticity: sequelae and burden on stroke survivors and caregivers. Neurology. 2013;80(3 Suppl 2):S45–52.

[17] Urban PP, Wolf T, Uebele M, Marx JJ, Vogt T, Stoeter P, et al. Occurrence and clinical predictors of spasticity after ischemic stroke. Stroke. 2010;41(9):2016–20.

[18] Sheean G, Lannin NA, Turner-Stokes L, Rawicki B, Snow BJ. Botulinum toxin assessment, intervention and after-care for upper limb hypertonicity in adults: international consensus statement. Eur J Neurol. 2010;17(Suppl 2):74–93.

[19] Sunnerhagen KS, Olver J, Francisco GE. Assessing and treating functional impairment in poststroke spasticity. Neurology. 2013;80(3 Suppl 2):S35–44.

[20] Byrnes ML, Thickbroom GW, Wilson SA, Sacco P, Shipman JM, Stell R, et al. The corticomotor representation of upper limb muscles in writer's cramp and changes following botulinum toxin injection. Brain. 1998;121(5):977–88.

[21] Kaňovský P, Streitová H, Dufek J, Znojil V, Daniel P, Rektor I. Change in lateralization of the P22/N30 cortical component of median nerve somatosensory evoked potentials

in patients with cervical dystonia after successful treatment with botulinum toxin A. Mov Disord. 1998;13(1):108–17.

[22] Gilio F, Currà A, Lorenzano C, Modugno N, Manfredi M, Berardelli A. Effects of botulinum toxin type A on intracortical inhibition in patients with dystonia. Ann Neurol. 2000;48(1):20–6.

[23] Kaňovský P, Bares M, Streitová H, Klajblová H, Daniel P, Rektor I. Abnormalities of cortical excitability and cortical inhibition in cervical dystonia Evidence from somatosensory evoked potentials and paired transcranial magnetic stimulation recordings. J Neurol. 2003;250(1):42–50.

[24] Kaňovský P, Rosales RL. Debunking the pathophysiological puzzle of dystonia--with special reference to botulinum toxin therapy. Parkinsonism Relat Disord. 2011;17(Suppl 1):S11–14.

[25] Opavský R, Hluštík P, Otruba P, Kaňovský P. Sensorimotor network in cervical dystonia and the effect of botulinum toxin treatment: a functional MRI study. J Neurol Sci. 2011;306(1–2):71–5.

[26] Opavský R, Hluštík P, Otruba P, Kaňovský P. Somatosensory cortical activation in cervical dystonia and its modulation with botulinum toxin: an fMRI study. Int J Neurosci. 2012;122(1):45–52.

[27] Johansen-Berg H, Dawes H, Guy C, Smith SM, Wade DT, Matthews PM. Correlation between motor improvements and altered fMRI activity after rehabilitative therapy. Brain. 2002;125(Pt 12):2731–42.

[28] Pundik S, Falchook AD, McCabe J, Litinas K, Daly JJ. Functional Brain Correlates of Upper Limb Spasticity and Its Mitigation following Rehabilitation in Chronic Stroke Survivors. Stroke Res Treat. 2014;2014:306325.

[29] Šenkárová Z, Hlustík P, Otruba P, Herzig R, Kanovský P. Modulation of cortical activity in patients suffering from upper arm spasticity following stroke and treated with botulinum toxin A: an fMRI study. J Neuroimaging. 2010;20(1):9–15.

[30] Tomášová Z, Hluštík P, Král M, Otruba P, Herzig R, Krobot A, et al. Cortical activation changes in patients suffering from post-stroke arm spasticity and treated with botulinum toxin A. J Neuroimaging. 2013;23(3):337–44.

[31] Manganotti P, Acler M, Formaggio E, Avesani M, Milanese F, Baraldo A, et al. Changes in cerebral activity after decreased upper-limb hypertonus: an EMG-fMRI study. Magn Reson Imaging. 2010;28(5):646–52.

[32] Veverka T, Hluštík P, Tomášová Z, Hok P, Otruba P, Král M, et al. BoNT-A related changes of cortical activity in patients suffering from severe hand paralysis with arm spasticity following ischemic stroke. J Neurol Sci. 2012;319(1-2): 89–95.

[33] Binkofski F, Buccino G. Motor functions of the Broca's region. Brain Lang. 2004;89(2):362–9.

[34] Diserens K, Ruegg D, Kleiser R, Hyde S, Perret N, Vuadens P, et al. Effect of repetitive arm cycling following botulinum toxin injection for poststroke spasticity: evidence from FMRI. Neurorehabil Neural Repair. 2010;24(8):753–62.

[35] Bergfeldt U, Jonsson T, Bergfeldt L, Julin P. Cortical activation changes and improved motor function in stroke patients after focal spasticity therapy—an interventional study applying repeated fMRI. BMC Neurol. 2015;15:52.

[36] Veverka T, Hluštík P, Hok P, Otruba P, Zapletalová J, Tüdös Z, et al. Sensorimotor modulation by botulinum toxin A in post-stroke arm spasticity: Passive hand movement. J Neurol Sci. 2016;362:14–20.

[37] Weiller C, Jüptner M, Fellows S, Rijntjes M, Leonhardt G, Kiebel S, et al. Brain representation of active and passive movements. Neuroimage. 1996;4(2):105–10.

[38] Johnson EA. Clostridial toxins as therapeutic agents: benefits of nature's most toxic proteins. Annu Rev Microbiol. 1999;53:551–75.

[39] Rossetto O, Morbiato L, Caccin P, Rigoni M, Montecucco C. Presynaptic enzymatic neurotoxins. J Neurochem. 2006;97(6):1534–45.

[40] Hallett M, Glocker FX, Deuschl G. Mechanism of action of botulinum toxin. Ann Neurol. 1994;36(3):449–50.

[41] Abbruzzese G, Berardelli A. Neurophysiological effects of botulinum toxin type A. Neurotox Res. 2006;9(2–3):109–14.

[42] Gelb DJ, Yoshimura DM, Olney RK, Lowenstein DH, Aminoff MJ. Change in pattern of muscle activity following botulinum toxin injections for torticollis. Ann Neurol. 1991;29(4):370–6.

[43] Deuschl G, Heinen F, Kleedorfer B, Wagner M, Lücking CH, Poewe W. Clinical and polymyographic investigation of spasmodic torticollis. J Neurol. 1992;239(1):9–15.

[44] Marin C, Martí MJ, Tolosa E, Alvarez R, Montserrat LL, Santamaria J. Modification of muscle activity after BOTOX injections in spasmodic torticollis. Ann Neurol. 1992;32(3):411–2.

[45] Marin C, Martí MJ, Tolosa E, Alvarez R, Montserrat L, Santamaria J. Muscle activity changes in spasmodic torticollis after botulinum toxin treatment. Eur J Neurol. 1995;1(3):243–7.

[46] Kaňovský P, Dufek J, Halačková H, Rektor I. Change in the pattern of cervical dystonia might be the cause of benefit loss during botulinum toxin treatment. Eur J Neurol. 1997;4(1):79–84.

http://dx.doi.org/10.5772/64763

[47] Abbruzzese G, Marchese R, Buccolieri A, Gasparetto B, Trompetto C. Abnormalities of sensorimotor integration in focal dystonia: a transcranial magnetic stimulation study. Brain. 2001;124(Pt 3):537–45.

[48] Frasson E, Priori A, Bertolasi L, Mauguière F, Fiaschi A, Tinazzi M. Somatosensory disinhibition in dystonia. Mov Disord. 2001;16(4):674–82.

[49] Meunier S, Garnero L, Ducorps A, Mazières L, Lehéricy S, Du Montcel ST, et al. Human brain mapping in dystonia reveals both endophenotypic traits and adaptive reorganization. Ann Neurol. 2001;50(4):521–7.

[50] Quartarone A, Rizzo V, Bagnato S, Morgante F, Sant'Angelo A, Romano M, et al. Homeostatic-like plasticity of the primary motor hand area is impaired in focal hand dystonia. Brain. 2005;128(Pt 8):1943–50.

Chapter 3

How does Recent Understanding of Molecular Mechanisms in Botulinum Toxin Impact Therapy?

Nutan Sharma

Additional information is available at the end of the chapter

http://dx.doi.org/10.5772/66696

Abstract

Botulinum toxin, one of the most lethal toxins identified, is also used as a therapeutic agent for a variety of human conditions. The history of the discovery of botulinum toxin, an understanding of its function at the molecular level and its development into a therapeutic reagent are instructive and allow the reader to build a conceptual framework around which to understand its current therapeutic uses and consider potential further uses of botulinum toxin.

Keywords: botulinum toxin, development, biochemistry, molecular biology, therapeutics

1. History of botulinum toxin

In 1817, Justinus Kerner published for the first time a report on a lethal case of food poisoning from eating spoiled sausages. He proposed that a biological poison was the culprit [1]. Subsequently, Dr. Kerner published two monographs of his observations on "sausage poisoning." In 1820, he described 76 cases in great detail [2]. Two years later, he described another 155 cases and also provided the first accurate and detailed description of the neuromuscular symptoms of botulism [3]. Dr. Kerner also conducted experiments in animals: cats, rabbits and birds that were given "spoiled sausage extracts." Dr. Kerner observed that motor neurons were affected in the treated animals, resulting in paralysis, while brain and sensory neurons were largely unchanged. Dr. Kerner went so far as to ingest botulinum neurotoxin (BoNT) himself and record the effects. He experienced difficulty in controlling his eyes, constipation and dryness in both the palms of his hands and soles of his feet [1]. From his clinical observations and animal experiments, Dr. Kerner concluded that this biological toxin could be used for medical purposes in those with disease resulting from an overly excited nervous system, such as St. Vitus's dance (chorea), excessive mucous production, or excessive sweating.

In 1897, Emile Pierre van Ermengem identified and cultured the bacteria that produced botulinum toxin. After an outbreak of botulism that resulted from the ingestion of contaminated ham, van Ermengem associated the growth of anaerobic bacteria on the meat with botulism [4, 5]. He isolated and cultured the anaerobic bacteria and then prepared a toxin extract. He performed and described many animal experiments and correctly deduced that the bacteria themselves do not cause food-borne botulism, but rather produce a toxin that after ingestion causes the illness. Subsequently, the toxin was named botulinum neurotoxin (BoNT) and the bacteria that produce it were named *Clostridium botulinum*. In 1949, Burgen and colleagues demonstrated that BoNT acts by blocking the release of acetylcholine at the neuromuscular junction [6].

2. Molecular biology and biochemistry

To date, seven different serotypes of BoNT have been identified, designated A–G. Four of the BoNT serotypes (A, B, E and F) cause human botulism, a neuroparalytic disease that may be fatal without proper diagnosis and treatment [7]. Using the tools of molecular biology, the serotypes have been studied in greater detail in order to understand their potential lethality and identify those serotypes with greater therapeutic and less lethal effect.

The genes encoding the BoNT serotypes have been isolated from multiple strains of *C. botulinum*. Six of the serotypes have several subtypes that differ significantly at the amino acid level [8–11]. Sequence comparison has identified eight different subtypes of BoNT/A, designated A1–A8 that vary in amino acid sequence. Similarly, sequence comparison has identified seven different subtypes of BoNT/B [12]. While these data were obtained to help with future identification of the source of botulism outbreaks, the sequence differences may be exploited to develop safer therapeutic forms of BoNT.

Each BoNT isoform is synthesized as a single, inactive polypeptide with a molecular mass of approximately 150 kDa. The precursor protein is cleaved by proteases into a 50-kDa light chain (LC) and a 100-kDa heavy chain (HC) that are linked by a disulfide bridge. The toxicity of BoNT is mediated by four distinct steps: binding to the presynaptic neuron, internalization in the neuron, translocation of the LC into the cytosol and proteolytic cleavage of a target protein. The initial binding sites of BoNT on nerve cells are polysialogangliosides [13–15]. While the exact mechanism is unknown, current models suggest that the polysialogangliosides serve to bring the BoNT out of the fluid phase and into the plane of the cell membrane. The carboxyl terminal of the HC chain of the BoNT then mediates binding to the exterior cell surface, presumably via an as-yet unidentified protein receptor [16]. Endocytosis, a temperature- and energy-dependent process, results in internalized BoNT that resides in a vesicle within the cytoplasm. Translocation then begins with the acidification of the vesicle lumen. Acidification results in conformational changes in the BoNT protein that facilitate translocation across the vesicle membrane and into the cytosol. During translocation, the disulfide bond between the heavy and light chains is broken and the two chains separate [11, 17]. The unbound LC is then able to express its catalytic activity in the cytosol [17, 18].

The LC portion of the BoNT peptide cleaves specific target proteins of the SNARE complex. BoNT/A and BoNT/E cleave the plasma membrane-associated protein SNAP-25 (synaptosome-associated protein of 25 kDa), whereas BoNT types B, D, F and G cleave synaptobrevin, a vesicle-associated membrane protein, also known as VAMP. The SNARE complex is composed of multiple members of a large protein super family that plays an essential role in the fusion of vesicles to their target membrane. In neurons, the SNARE complex is critical in mediating the docking of synaptic vesicles with the presynaptic membrane [19–21]. Thus, cleavage of a critical protein in the SNARE complex results in decreased vesicle fusion with the presynaptic membrane. The result is reduced neurotransmission. When BoNT is injected into the skeletal muscle, in the vicinity of the neuromuscular junction, the presynaptic neuron is unable to release acetylcholine. The result is a decreased stimulus indicating that the muscle should contract and muscle relaxation ensues.

3. Therapeutic development

It was not until the mid-twentieth century that scientists developed standardized methods for the production and stabilization of BoNT serotype A (BoNT/A) [22–28]. Thanks to these efforts, Alan Scott was then able to demonstrate that BoNT/A could treat strabismus in monkeys by injecting toxin into their extra ocular muscles [29]. This was followed by successful trials in humans with strabismus [30]. Since the 1980s, BoNT/A has been used to treat neuromuscular hyperactivity disorders, as first conceived by Justinus Kerner in the early nineteenth century. The original batch of BoNT/A, purified for human use, was registered under the name Oculinum. In 1991, the company and 125 mg of the originally purified BoNT/A were sold to Allergan (Irvine, CA). The drug was given the trade name of Botox and the initial 125 mg of toxin was the exclusive source of drug until 1998, when a continuous manufacturing process was put into production [31].

Currently, BoNT serotypes A1 and B are available for therapeutic use. The toxin is injected into the immediate vicinity of nerve endings for a host of therapeutic purposes, including the alleviation of focal dystonia, spasticity, hyperhidrosis, prophylactic migraine treatment and reduction of glabellar lines. In all of these conditions, the interruption of cholinergic neurotransmission results in the desired therapeutic effect. For the treatment of dystonia or spasticity, for example, BoNT/A has been shown to have effects on both extrafusal fibers, which compose skeletal muscle and are innervated by acetylcholine released at the neuromuscular junction and intrafusal fibers, which are innervated by acetylcholine released by gamma motor neurons at contractile ends and thus serve as a sensory proprioceptor [32]. Extrafusal fibers are integral to muscle contraction and thus are affected in focal dystonia. Intrafusal fibers monitor the velocity of a muscle stretch and thus play a role in mediating skeletal muscle spasticity. By reducing cholinergic transmission to extrafusal and intrafusal fibers, both dystonia and spasticity can be reduced. For the treatment of hyperhidrosis, intradermal injection of BoNT/A in the axilla results in reduced cholinergic neurotransmission from the sympathetic fibers that innervate the eccrine glands. For the prophylactic treatment of chronic migraine, the mechanism by which the intramuscular injection of BoNT/A, following a fixed pattern of injection sites, results in reduced headache frequency is unknown.

Three different brands of BoNT/A1 are available in the United States: onabotulinum toxinA (Botox), incobotulinum toxinA (Xeomin) and Abobotulinum toxinA (Dysport). In addition, one form of BoNT/B is available, rimabotulinum toxinB (Myobloc). There are a limited number of comparative studies between the different brands. However, two distinct studies, comparing the effectiveness of onabotulinum toxinA to rimabotulinum toxinB in cervical dystonia subjects, indicate that both serotypes are equally efficacious with a possibly slightly longer duration of action in those treated with onabotulinum toxinA [33, 34]. Thus, in the treatment of cervical dystonia, differences between serotypes and subtypes of BoNT may not produce a significant difference in therapeutic effect. For the treatment of axillary hyperhidrosis, a recent study found that both onabotulinum toxinA and rimabotulinum toxinB were equal in the onset of action, the duration of action and therapeutic efficacy [35].

4. Future applications

With our more detailed knowledge of the mechanism of action of BoNT and better understanding of the mechanisms of various disease states, it is possible that the specificity and proteolytic activity of the various BoNT serotypes may be used for a wide variety of medical purposes. A recent publication demonstrated that modified BoNT may be targeted to inflammatory immune cells, disrupting the SNARE complex in those cells and resulting in the blockade of the release of inflammatory cytokine tumor necrosis factor [36]. In the future, the specificity of the HC portion of BoNT may be used to target a variety of agents to presynaptic cholinergic neurons. In addition, the HC portion of BoNT may be modified, to change its cellular target, to allow for the delivery of small molecules to other cell types.

Author details

Nutan Sharma

Address all correspondence to: nsharma@partners.org

Massachusetts General Hospital, Harvard Medical School, Boston, MA, USA

References

[1] Pellett S. Learning from the past: Historical aspects of bacterial toxins as pharmaceuticals. Curr Opin Microbiol. 2012;15:292–299.

[2] Kerner J. New Observations on the Occasional Occurrences in Wurtembrg of Fatal Poisoning Cases by Enjoying Smoked Sausages. Osiander; 1820.

[3] Kerner J. Grease Or Fatty Acid And Its Effects, A Surgery To Investigate The Substance Of Toxic Substance In Spoiled Deserts. Cotta; 1822

[4] van Ermengem E. Classics in infectious diseases. A new anaerobic bacillus and its relation to botulism. Rev Infect Dis. 1979;1:701–719.

[5] Ermengem E. On a new anaerobic bacillus and its relations to Botulism. Med Microbiol Immunol (Berl) 1897:1–56.

[6] Burgen AS, Dickens F, Zatman LJ. The action of botulinum toxin on the neuromuscular junction. J Physiol 1949;109:10–24.

[7] Arnon SS, Schechter R, Inglesby TV, Henderson DA, Bartlett JG, et al. Botulinum toxin as a biological weapon: medical and public health management. JAMA 2001;285:1059–1570.

[8] Arndt JW, Jacobson MJ, Abola EE, Forsyth CM, Tepp WH, et al. A structural perspective of the sequence variability within botulinum neurotoxin subtypes A1–A4. J Mol Biol. 2006;362:733–742.

[9] Hill KK, Smith TJ, Helma CH, Ticknor LO, Foley BT, et al. Genetic diversity among botulinum neurotoxin-producing clostridial strains. J Bacteriol. 2007;189:818–832.

[10] Johnson EA, Montecucco C: Botulism. In: Engel AG, editor, Handbook of Clinical Neurology. Elsevier; 2008. pp. 333–368.

[11] Montal M. Botulinum neurotoxin: a marvel of protein design. Annu Rev Biochem. 2010;79:591–617.

[12] Kalb SR, Baudys J, Rees JC, Smith TJ, Smith LA, et al. De Novo subtype and strain identification of botulinum neurotoxin type B through toxin proteomics. Anal Bioanal Chem. 2012;403: 215–226.

[13] Schiavo G, Matteoli M, Montecucco C. Neurotoxins affecting neuroexocytosis. Physiol Rev. 2000;80:717–766.

[14] Montecucco C, Rossetto O, Schiavo G. Presynaptic receptor arrays for clostridial neurotoxins. Trends Microbiol. 2004;12:442–446.

[15] Simpson L. The life history of a botulinum toxin molecule. Toxicon. 2013;68:40–59.

[16] Swaminathan S. Molecular structures and functional relationships in clostridial neurotoxins. FEBS. 2011;278:4467–4485. doi:10.1111/j.1742-4658.2011.08183.x

[17] Fischer A, Montal M. Crucial role of the disulfide bridge between botulinum neurotoxin light and heavy chains in protease translocation across membranes. J Biol Chem. 2007;282:29604–29611.

[18] Koriazova LK, Montal M. Translocation of botulinum neurotoxin light chain protease through the heavy chain channel. Nat Struc Biol. 2003;10:13–18.

[19] Sudhof TC, Rothman JE. Membrane fusion: grappling with SNARE and SM proteins. Science. 2009;323:474–77.

[20] Sutton RB, Fasshauer D, Jahn R, Brunger AT. Crystal structure of a SNARE complex involved in synaptic exocytosis at 2.4 Å resolution. Nature. 1998;395:347–353.

[21] Weber T, Zemelman BV, McNew JA, Westermann B, Gmachl M, et al. SNAREpins: minimal machinery for membrane fusion. Cell. 1998;92:759–772.

[22] Boor AK, Tresselt HB, Schantz EJ. Effects of salts and colloids on potency of botulinum toxin. Proc Soc Exp Biol Med. 1955;89:270–272.

[23] Buehler HJ, Schantz EJ, Lamanna C. The elemental and amino acid composition of crystalline Clostridium botulinum type A toxin. J Biol Chem. 1947;169:295–302.

[24] Lamanna C, Spero L, Schantz EJ. Dependence of time to death on molecular size of botulinum toxin. Infect Immun. 1970;1:423–424.

[25] Schantz EJ. Some chemical and physical properties of Clostridium botulinum toxins in culture. Jpn J Microbiol. 1967;11:380–383.

[26] Schantz EJ, Stefanye D, Spero L. Observations on the fluorescence and toxicity of botulinum toxin. J Biol Chem. 1960;235:3489–3491.

[27] Stefanye D, Schantz EJ, Spero L. Amino acid composition of crystalline botulinum toxin, type A. J Bacteriol. 1967;94:277–278.

[28] Weil L, Seibles TS, Spero L, Schantz EJ. Photooxidation of crystalline Clostridium botulinum type A toxin in the presence of methylene blue. Arch Biochem Biophys. 1957;68:308–313.

[29] Scott AB, Rosenbaum A, Collins CC. Pharmacologic weakening of extraocular muscles. Invest Ophthalmol. 1973;12:924–927.

[30] Scott AB. Botulinum toxin injection into extraocular muscles as an alternative to strabismus surgery. J Pediatr Ophthalmol Strabismus. 1980;17:21–25.

[31] Dressler D. Botulinum toxin drugs: brief history and outlook. J Neural Transm. 2016;123:277–279.

[32] Rosales RL, Arimura K, Takenaga S, Osame M. Extrafusal and intrafusal muscle effects in experimental botulinum toxin-A injection. Muscle Nerve. 1996;19:488–4960.

[33] Comella CL, Jankovic J, Shannon KM, Tsui J, et al. Comparison of botulinum toxin serotypes A and B for the treatment of cervical dystonia. Neurology. 2005;65:1423–1429.

[34] Pappert EJ, Germanson T, Myobloc/Neurobloc European Cervical Dystonia Study Group. Botulinum toxin type B vs. type A in toxin-naïve patients with cervical dystonia: Randomized, double-blind noninferiority trial. Mov Disord. 2008;23:510–517.

[35] An JS, Hyun Won C, Si Han J, Park HS, Seo KK, Comparison of onabotulinum toxinA and rimabotulinumtoxinB for the treatment of axillary hyperhidrosis. Dermatol Surg. 2015;41:960–967.

[36] Yeh FL, Zhu Y, Tepp WH, Johnson EA, Bertics PJ, Chapman ER. Retargeted clostridial neurotoxins as novel agents for treating chronic diseases. Biochemistry. 2011;50:10419–10421. doi: 10.1021/bi201490t.

Chapter 4

Clinical Relevance of Immunoresistance to Botulinum Therapy

Jürgen Frevert and Dirk Dressler

Additional information is available at the end of the chapter

http://dx.doi.org/10.5772/64566

Abstract

Because botulinum toxin is a bacterial antigen, the therapy with this biological bears the risk that the formation of antibodies is elicited which can neutralize the neurotoxin. Several factors have an impact on this immune response. There are (unknown) patient-related factors but also the dose, the injection interval and the purity of the product play a role in the formation of antibodies. Several assays to detect antibodies are available; immunological assays such as FIA (fluorescence immunoassay) and ELISA, function assays such as MPA (mouse protection assay) and HDA (hemidiaphragm assay), clinical assays such as the EDB assay (extensor digitorum brevis assay), and SCM assay (sternocleidomastoid) which have different sensitivities. Clinical studies with different BoNT/A products demonstrate that the rate of antibody formation is low. Important for the physician is whether the antibody formation has an impact on the responsiveness of the patient. Not all patients with positive sera are nonresponders. The antibody titer is certainly important which might not be high enough to neutralize the injected dose completely but the titer might increase during further treatment with the neurotoxin leading to complete nonresponse. To avoid the formation of antibodies, the lowest dose necessary for the patient should be injected keeping the longest acceptable injection interval.

Keywords: botulinum neurotoxin, neutralizing antibodies, secondary nonresponse, immunogenicity, treatment failure

1. Introduction

Cervical dystonia (CD) is a chronic disease lasting for the rest of a patient's life and requires a lifelong treatment. Injection of botulinum neurotoxin type A (BoNT/A) is recommended by the

European Federation of Neurological Societies (EFNS) as the first line treatment for primary crandial and cervical dystonia [1]. Currently, three products are approved for medical use in Western markets, and all are approved by the FDA: onabotulinumtoxin A (ONA; Botox/ Vistabel®, Allergan Inc., Irvine, CA), abobotulinumtoxin A (ABO; Dysport®Ipsen, Paris, France), and incobotulinumtoxin A (INCO; Xeomin®, Merz Pharmaceuticals GmbH, Frankfurt Germany). The efficacy and safety of these three commercially available BoNT/A preparations have been well established with level A recommendations. Botulinum toxin products are also successfully applied in a broad range of medical indications in the field of other movement disorders (e.g., spasticity, blepharospasm); urological disorders (e.g., overactive bladder) as well as aesthetic indications. This review will focus on clinical studies in CD and spasticity.

There are also several botulinum toxin products originating and approved in Asian countries: in Korea Neuronox (Mecytox Inc), Nabota (Daewong Inc.), Botulax (Hugel Inc.), and from China BTXA or Lantox (Lanzou Institute) with a drug substance similar to ONA but with a different manufacturing process and formulation. Studies conducted with these products will not be further discussed in this chapter. The only approved botulinum toxin type B product (BoNT/B) is Myobloc/Neurobloc (rimabotulinumtoxinB, RIMA, US World Meds, Lousiville, KY). BoNT/B can be used when there is resistance to BoNT/A.

The molecular composition and mechanism of action of BoNTs are described in numerous reviews and are only briefly summarized here [2, 3]. The active moiety in all BoNT/A products is the neurotoxin, a 1296 amino acid long protein with a relatively high molecular weight of 150 kD [3, 4]. BoNT/A is synthesized by the anaerobic bacterium *Clostridium botulinum* as a single-chain protein, which is cleaved into two subunits by a clostridial protease resulting in two subunits, a heavy chain and a light chain, linked by a disulphide bridge. The C-terminal domain of the heavy chain binds highly specifically to receptor molecules on the presynaptic membrane of cholinergic neurons. The heavy chain has two binding domains, one for special glycolipids (GT1b) and the other for a protein receptor called SV2 [5]. The receptor-bound BoNT is taken up into the nerve cell by endocytosis. The second domain of the heavy chain called translocation domain then facilitates the release of the light chain out of the endocytotic vesicle into the cytosol of the neuron. The smaller subunit, the light chain, is a highly specific protease which cleaves a neuronal protein, the so-called SNARE protein, SNAP25, required for the secretion of acetylcholine. Cleaved SNAP25 has lost its ability to function in the secretory process. As a result, the acetylcholine-containing secretory vesicle cannot fuse with the presynaptic membrane, acetylcholine is not secreted, and so the muscle cell is no longer activated and becomes paralyzed [6]. By this mechanism, BoNT blocks cholinergic muscular innervation of striated and smooth muscles as well as the cholinergic innervation of exocrine glands (sweat gland, saliva gland). The mode of action is identical for all BoNT/A products. Other BoNT serotypes act in a similar way but their receptor molecules, and substrates are different, for example, BoNT/B, the active substance in RIMA, cleaves a SNARE protein called VAMP [4].

As a bacterial protein, botulinum toxin is a foreign protein to the host immune system, that is, per se an antigen and bears, therefore, the risk to elicit the formation of antibodies particularly because botulinum toxin has to be applied repeatedly after the therapeutic effect has waned off. The formation of antibodies against the protein can lead to secondary treatment failure, to nonresponse (secondary nonresponse, SNR), that is, to the termination of the therapy.

This review will discuss the formation of neutralizing antibodies against botulinum toxin particularly in the treatment of CD and spasticity regarding the immunogenicity of this highly efficacious protein and its clinical implications.

2. Development of antibodies against botulinum neurotoxin and secondary nonresponse

2.1. Immunogenicity of botulinum toxin products

All products contain the 150 kD neurotoxin as the active principle, a foreign protein to the human immune system. This protein is produced by clostridia and is embedded into a complex formed with other bacterial proteins, the so-called complexing proteins or neurotoxin-associated proteins (NAPs) [7]. Some of these proteins are biologically active. They belong to lectins and bind to glycoproteins or glycolipids on cell membranes [8]. They are called hemagglutinins with respect to their capability to agglutinate red blood cells. This specific activity is certainly not required in the treatment of movement disorders. The hemagglutinins are rather necessary in the process of oral intoxication with the toxin. Thus, the complexing proteins have no function in the therapy with botulinum toxin.

Therapeutic proteins which are administered repeatedly can elicit the formation of antibodies, even when these proteins originate from human sources [9]. These antibodies can lead to loss of efficacy [9]. As botulinum toxin products contain bacterial proteins and are administered repeatedly, they have an even higher risk to stimulate the formation of antibodies directed against the neurotoxin, and/or in the case of ONA and ABO against the complexing proteins [10]. In principal antibodies against the active substance will interfere with the therapy. Depending on the antibody titer, it can lead to partial therapy failure or—if the antibody titer is high enough—to a complete treatment failure or secondary nonresponse [11]. In general, partial treatment failure precedes complete treatment failure as demonstrated in a (small) clinical study with 27 patients. Twenty two of these patients showed partial treatment failure. Before comlete nonresponse occurred [12]. It is obvious that antibodies directed against the binding domain of the neurotoxin heavy chain will inhibit the binding of the neurotoxin to the neuron or inhibit the translocation and consequently neutralize the activity [13, 14]. Antibodies directed against the enzymatic domain (light chain) can also inhibit the neurotoxin's activity because of steric hindrance of the translocation process [13].

Apart from patient-related factors (sensitivity of the patient's immune system), several product-related factors may influence the immunogenicity of biological proteins (see **Table 1**). In case of BoNT products, the manufacturing process, the antigenic protein load, and the presence of complexing proteins contribute to the immune response but treatment-related factors, for example, the interval between injections, booster injections, and prior exposure may also be involved. The role the protein load and treatment intervals play in the process of antibody formation is convincingly demonstrated by the first generation of ONA. It contained 10 times more antigenic protein (50 ng of clostridial protein) than the current formulation. Consequently, it generated a high rate of antibody formation and secondary nonresponders [15, 16]. Therefore, physicians were advised to keep the intervals between single treatments as long as acceptable for the patient to prevent the formation of antibodies [17]. The amount of neurotoxin protein in ONA has since been markedly reduced to 5 ng clostridial protein, (corresponding to 0.83 ng neurotoxin protein) leading to a marked decrease in antibody formation [18] (see further discussion in Section 2.3.1).

According to CHMP guideline EMEA/CHMP/BMWP/14327/2006; 2008
Factors that may influence the development of an immune response against a therapeutic protein
• Patient and disease-related factors
• Genetic factors modulating the immune response
• Genetic factors related to a gene defect
• Age
• Disease-related factors
• Concomitant treatment
• Duration, route of administration, treatment modalities
• Previous exposure to similar or related proteins
Product-related factors of immunogenicity
• Protein structure
• Formulation
• Aggregation and adduct formation
• Impurities

Table 1. Factors influencing immunogenic response.

Complexing proteins do not play a role in the mechanism of action of BoNT once it has reached body fluids; thus, antibodies directed against these proteins cannot block the activity of BoNT, they cannot neutralize the neurotoxin. It has been reported that approximately 50% of patients (treated for a therapeutic indication) develop antibodies against the complexing proteins without therapeutic consequences [19]. From this standpoint, complexing proteins are just inert proteins without any effects on BoNT therapy. However, new data suggest that this might not be the case. A growing body of evidence shows that complexing proteins can interact with the host immune system and, therefore, be clinically relevant [20].

To produce antibodies, the immune system needs to be activated. Not only the antigen has to be present, but also an activating signal [21]. The first cells that recognize the antigen (i.e., BoNT) are dendritic cells. These cells present the antigen to T-lymphocytes. These lymphocytes are then activated by cytokines secreted by the dendritic cells. The activated T-lymphocytes subsequently activate B-lymphocytes which produce the antibodies [21]. Dendritic cells have exposed pattern recognition receptors (toll-like receptors), which react with different bacterial products such as bacterial DNA, parts of the bacterial cell wall, and bacterial proteins such as flagellin and hemagglutinins [21]. The latter are known to act as adjuvants, which bind to and activate dendritic cells [22].

The first step of the binding to immune cells has been demonstrated by analyzing the interaction of the BoNT complex, and the purified BoNT, free from complexing proteins, with lymphoblasts, fibroblasts and a human neuroblastoma cell line (as a control) [20]. It was shown that both the complexing proteins and the BoNT complex reacted with the lymphoblasts, in contrast to the pure BoNT [20]. And moreover, whereas the purified BoNT did not influence the release of inflammatory cytokines, BoNT complex and the complexing proteins lead to a dramatic increase in release [20]. Thus, the complexing proteins can affect the formation of antibodies against BoNT by stimulating dendritic cells.

2.2. Assays to detect antibodies against botulinum neurotoxin

The simplest way assays to detect antibodies are immunoassay-based procedures such as enzyme-linked immunosorbent assay (ELISA), the fluorescence immunoassay (FIA), and the immunoprecipitation assay [23]. These assays are often used in clinical studies to screen sera of a large patient population. Positive samples are then further evaluated in functional assays because immunassays cannot discriminate between neutralizing and non neutralizing antibodies; they only detect antibodies that bind to the antigen, botulinum neurotoxin. Whether these antibodies inhibit the activity of the neurotoxin cannot be assessed with these assays, and therefore, the assay results cannot be correlated with therapeutic response.

A method used for the detection of BoNT neutralizing antibodies must test the function of each domain of the neurotoxin: binding, translocation, as well as the catalytic (proteolytic) activity of the light chain in one assay or in a set of assays, because antibodies can be directed against only one domain and its affinity might not be high enough to inhibit the binding to the neuronal receptor or prevent the uptake of the neurotoxin into the nerve cell. If a single functional assay is applied, it should be based on intact cellular systems. The easiest test is the mouse protection assay (MPA). Mice are treated with increasing doses of BoNT and their survival rate is determined. This assay is presently considered the gold standard because the median lethal dose (MLD) can be determined very accurately [24]. The MLD increases when BoNT antibodies are present. By means of a calibration curve, based upon standard antibody titers, titers in patients' sera can be calculated. However, exact titers determined with the MPA are rarely published. Often the MPA assay is carried out by injecting a mixture of a LD100 dose of the toxin with the serum of a respective patient into five mice. If all mice survive, the serum is antibody-positive [18]. The correlation between the MPA and clinical responsiveness was investigated in an early study with 51 patients (34 nonresponder and 17 responder [25]); the specificity of the assay was high (100%), no patient with a negative titer in the MPA showed a clinical nonresponse. A disadvantage of the MPA is its low sensitivity. Only half of the patients with nonresponse showed a positive MPA result. This result may be explained by the fact that the detection limit of the assay is too high [25] or the nonresponse might be caused by non-immunological factors.

The MPA has many disadvantages. The test is costly, requires several days before it can be evaluated and exposes the test animals to prolonged agony including respiratory failure. Since the endpoint of the test is the paralysis of the respiratory muscle, a truncated version of the test is represented by an isolated nerve muscle, the phrenic-hemidiaphragm preparation (mouse hemidiaphragm assay; HDA). In this assay, the serum of the patient is incubated with a fixed amount of the neurotoxin followed by the measurement of the effect on the contraction amplitude of an indirectly stimulated mouse hemidiaphragm mounted into an organ bath [26]. This assay is quantitative and highly sensitive, about 25 times more sensitive than the MPA [27].

A disadvantage of the assay is that a high amount of patient's serum is required (4.0 mL) so that in most cases, the serum sample is only determined once.

Because cell-based assays (CBA) are now approved to replace the LD50 assay, the CBA could also be adapted to determine antibodies.

All these functional assays analyze the antibody titer in sera and not in the muscle in which the neurotoxin is applied and potentially neutralized. The antibody titer in sera and in muscles must not necessarily be identical. This fact could explain why patient with an antibody titer still respond to neurotoxin. To circumvent this disadvantage, clinical assays were developed that measure—indirectly—the inhibitory activity of antibodies in muscles. These include the extensor digitorum brevis test (EDB) [28] the unilaterally brow injection test (UBI) [29], the sternocleidomastoid test SCM [30], and the sudomotor sweat test [31]. They are generally not quantitative (results are "positive" or "negative" based on the judgment of the investigator) and do not determine the antibody titer directly but it's clinical effect and principally show a satisfactory correlation with the responsiveness of the patient, which means that they do not provide assay-positive results for patients who are still sensitive to botulinum toxin therapy. Although very valuable for the clinical practice these assays are usually not applied in large clinical studies because patients have to be reinjected when nonresponse occurred and judged in a visit after additional days.

2.3. Factors which determine the formation of antibodies

The CHMP guideline on immunogenicity assessment of biotechnology-derived therapeutic proteins lists factors, which determine the formation of antibodies in patients (**Table 1**) [32]; some of them are patient related and some are based on the product and its application. Until today, no investigations are published why patients develop antibodies against botulinum neurotoxins. It is unclear whether for instance the specific HLA repertoire of a patient favors the formation of antibodies or other patient-related (e.g. genetic) factors. There could be a higher incidence of antibody formation in children as found in an early study, in which 35 of 110 treated children developed an antibody titer and became secondary nonresponder [33]. More research, however, is needed to confirm this risk factor. In the following, some factors related to the products and clinical procedures are discussed.

2.3.1. Dose of the neurotoxin

In general, the dose of an antigen determines the formation of antibodies: a higher dose bears a higher risk of antibody formation. But so far, there is no defined threshold below which no antibodies are produced.

The first approved botulinum toxin product (ONA) contained a high amount of the neurotoxin complex: 25 ng (100 U) corresponding to 4.2 ng of the neurotoxin protein because a high amount of neurotoxin (ca 80%) was inactivated during manufacturing. Up to 17% of the patients treated with this product developed antibodies [18, 34, 35]. Based on an improved manufacturing process in 1997, a new lot of ONA became available which contains a substantially lower amount of the botulinum toxin complex leading to an about sixfold decreased rate of antibody formation [18]. Nevertheless, there is still inactive neurotoxin present in ONA which could enhance the risk of antibody formation [36].

The dose of RIMA in the treatment of CD is about 50 times higher than the dose of INCO and ONA, which means that a markedly higher amount of antigen is injected (about 12 times more neurotoxin protein). In addition, about 30% of the neurotoxin is inactive (because it is not processed into heavy and light chain) [37]. Therefore, approximately between 35 and 44% of patients treated with RIMA develop antibodies against BONT/B [38].

Table 2 provides an overview over the different amounts of bacterial protein and neurotoxin protein injected in comparable doses. The differences between the products are obvious: the high amount of neurotoxin protein in RIMA seems to be responsible for the high percentage of antibody formation. One would expect that the product with the lowest amount of antigen bears lowest risk of antibody formation (see below).

Product	Dose	Amount of protein (ng)	Amount of neurotoxin protein (ng)
ABO*	250 U	2.17	1.62
INCO*	100 U	0.44	0,44
ONA*	100 U	5	0.73
RIMA**	5000 U	≈55	≈11

* Calculated from Ref. [36].
** Calculated from Ref. [37].

Table 2. Amount of neurotoxin protein (antigen) injected into patient.

A higher cumulative dose seems to correlate with a higher risk of antibody formation: in an early study, Jankovic and Schwartz observed that patients with a titer of neutralizing antibody were treated with a higher cumulative dose (1709 U ± 638 U over 2.5 years) than patients with a lower cumulative dose (1066 U ± 938 U over 2.4 years) [16]. Göschel et al. found a correlation between a high dose and a high proportion of antibody formation in patients treated with ONA and/or ABO, but only a small population of 28 patients was analyzed [19]. Some indications require a higher dose than other and, therefore, bear a higher risk of antibody formation. This was confirmed by Lange et al. who showed that in patients treated for CD and spasticity higher doses correlate with a high rate of antibody formation [27]. This is in accordance with another study with patients suffering from CD. The patients with SNR received a higher dose than the responders. Also these authors concluded that a higher dose is a risk factor for the development of antibodies [39].

2.3.2. Injection interval

A second injection after a short injection interval might act as a "booster" injection. Greene et al. observed that patients whose sera were positive in the MPA had been treated with markedly shorter injection intervals [17]. An evaluation of sera of secondary nonresponders treated with ABO and ONA demonstrated that patients treated within 1–2 months showed a higher proportion of antibody formation than patients with an injection interval of 4–13 months [27]. Thus, a short treatment interval seems to correlate with a higher risk of antibody formation and secondary nonresponse. Greene et al. suggested to inject as infrequently as possible ideally no more frequently than 3 months [16]. This procedure is still standard clinical practice. In the prescribing information of all products, it is recommended not to reinject earlier than 12 weeks. Unfortunately, this interval is not adequate for all patients, some require an earlier treatment because of termination of the therapeutic effect. In a long-term prospective CD study, it was demonstrated that 22.5% of the patients reinjected with INCO <10 weeks and 24.6% between 10 and 12 weeks did not develop antibodies [40]. Although more long-term studies are required, the strict adherence to an injection interval of 12 weeks seems to be obsolete at least for INCO.

2.4. Antibody formation and secondary nonresponse in clinical studies

Generally, a two tier approach is used in clinical studies to identify patients with neutralizing antibodies: screening with an immunoassay and confirmation of positive results with a functional assay. Data for antibody formation in clinical studies cannot really be compared because the applied assays have a markedly different sensitivity, the mouse protection assay is at least 5 times (or even 25 times [27]) less sensitive as the mouse hemidiaphragm assay. In addition, there is no published information about the validation of the assays particularly concerning sensitivity and specificity of the assay. In the most cases studies with ONA, ABO, and RIMA apply the MPA whereas in studies with INCO only the HDA is used for the detection of neutralizing antibodies.

In the following, results derived from clinical studies with the different products are summarized. Studies with ONA before 1997 (the "old Botox") will not be discussed because it is no longer on the market. A most recent overview over neutralizing antibody formation in clinical studies is presented by Fabbri et al. [41].

2.4.1. Cervical dystonia

2.4.1.1. OnabotulinumtoxinA

Brin et al. conducted an open-label long-term observational study with ONA in 326 neurotoxin naïve patients over a mean of 2.5 years [42]. They reported the formation of antibodies during the course of up to 15 treatment cycles in 4 patients (1.2%) resulting from a mouse protection assay. Three of these patients lost responsiveness. One of these patients was also antibody positive in a clinical assay (FTAT), and the other two patients were not tested [42]. In a comparison of the current ONA with the pre-1997 product, it was found that none of the 119 patient treated with the current ONA developed neutralizing antibodies by applying the MPA [16].

2.4.1.2. *AbobotulinumtoxinA*

In a randomized, placebo-controlled study with 116 patients Truong et al. found one patient with neutralizing antibodies in the MPA, but this patient still responded to ABO [43]. Coleman et al. reported that 3 patients out of 136 developed neutralizing antibodies as tested with the MPA (2.2%), and two of these patients still responded to the treatment [44]. In a long-term open-label study conducted by Kessler et al., 303 patients with CD were treated with ≥6 injections of ONA. Nine of 17 secondary nonresponders were antibody positive in MPA, HDA, or EDB [45]. The rate of antibody formation was calculated with 2.5% referring to a total of 357 patients (54 patients discontinued the study) [45]. Antibody positive patients were treated with higher doses in shorter intervals and had a higher number of "booster" injections. In a long-term study (10–12 years) conducted by Haussermann et al. Three patients out of 90 patients became nonresponder (3.3%) but were antibody negative in the HDA [46].

2.4.1.3. *IncobotulinumotoxinA*

In a placebo-controlled study, four out of 233 patients developed antibodies during the placebo-controlled phase of the trial, four in the open-label phase according to the testing in the HDA, and none of these patients became secondary nonresponder [47]. It has to be mentioned that the antibody-positive patients were treated with other products before the study so the antibody formation might be primed by the other products. No naïve patient developed antibodies. This was also demonstrated in other studies with INCO [28–50]. In an open-label study conducted by Benecke with 100 patients previously treated with ONA, ABO or RIMA, no patient developed antibodies or secondary nonresponse during treatment with INCO for up to 2 years [51]. No patient developed new neutralizing antibodies in a trial with 76 patients with CD based on testing with the HDA. Three patients had neutralizing antibodies at screening (prior to treatment with incobotulinumtoxinA), two of whom experienced no loss of treatment effect 4 weeks after repeated injections of INCO, while a third patient did experience a loss of treatment effect after the second and subsequent INCO injections [52].

2.4.1.4. *RimabotulinumtoxinB*

Jankovic et al. conducted a 42 months lasting observational study: Patients who were previously treated with BoNT/A and partly developed antibodies against BoNT/A were treated with RIMA [38]. According to results of the MPA, 34.4% of the patients developed antibodies against BoNT/B whereas the proportion of patients with antibodies against BoNT/A declined from 13 to 2.5% during the course of the study [38]. Also in this study, the development of immunoresistance correlated with the dose of toxin. The rate of antibody formation after treatment with RIMA was high in three long-term studies, 33.0, 42.0–44.0, and 28% over 2, 4 or 7 years, respectively) [53]. Remarkably, most of the patients who discontinued the study because of poor efficacy did not develop antibody, precise numbers were not given. The authors assume that the development of antibodies did not correlate with the lack of efficacy. In contrast, in a small study by Dressler and Bigalke, four of the nine patients treated with RIMA became resistant to the therapy and developed antibodies against BoNT/B as shown in the HDA [54].

2.4.2. *Upper limp spasticity*

2.4.2.1. *OnabotulinumtoxinA*

In a pooled analysis of three studies with 191 post-stroke spasticity patients, Yablon et al. reported the development of antibodies in one patient assessed with the MPA (0.5%) [55]. The patient did not respond to ONA at any time of the study. Elovic et al. reported one patient out of 224 developed neutralizing antibodies according to the MPA (0.45%) [56]. At the end of the study, this patient was a nonresponder who was also confirmed in a clinical assay (FTAT).

2.4.2.2. *AbobotulinumtoxinA*

Baktheit reported in the only published study that no patient developed neutralizing antibodies in an open-label trial with 41 patients with post-stroke spasticity [57]. There was no information about secondary nonresponse.

2.4.2.3. *IncobotulinumtoxinA*

Applying the HDA after FIA screening, no neutralizing antibody formation was observed in a study by Kanovsky et al. Seventy three patients were treated in a single cycle with INCO [58]. No patient showed secondary nonresponse. This was also observed in another trial with 47 patients with arm spasticity reported by Dressler et al: no patient of developed antibodies or secondary treatment failure [59].

2.4.2.4. *RimabotulinumtoxinB*

Brashear et al. did not find antibody formation in 10 patient treated with10,000 U of RIMA in a 16 week study followed by a 12 week open-label extension period [60]. Secondary nonresponse was not observed.

In conclusion, the studies demonstrate that the formation of antibodies after treatment with BoNT/A products based on MPA or HDA is low and only very weakly correlated with secondary nonresponse. Patients with neutralizing antibodies were not necessarily nonresponders, and not every nonresponder was antibody positive. But it cannot be excluded that the analyzed titer is too low to neutralize the amount of injected neurotoxin. Because the immune system was already stimulated, it can be speculated that the antibody titer will increase over time with further injections ("booster") of the antigen (neurotoxin) leading to secondary nonresponse when the titer is sufficiently high. Long-term studies are warranted to observe antibody titer development and therapeutic responsiveness of antibody positive and responsive patients. Complete therapy failure seems to be preceded by partial therapy failure characterized by a low antibody titer which is also characterized by a shorter duration of effect [61].

http://dx.doi.org/10.5772/64566

Secondary nonresponse is not only caused by the formation of neutralizing antibodies. Many patients nonresponsive to BoNT have no detectable antibody titer. Lange et al. analyzed sera of 503 patients treated with ABO or ONA with the HDA and showed that 224 patient's sera (44.5%) contained neutralizing antibodies [27]. Of course, it cannot be excluded that assay results were false negative (the assays were carried only once for each serum, there was not confirmatory assays applied) or the sensitivity of the HDA was too low to detect antibodies which neutralize BoNT after injection in the muscle. More plausible is that lack of response might be caused by other factors like inadequate dosing, failure to inject the appropriate muscle or change in the pattern of muscle hyperactivity and changes in the disease state. Other more subjective factors may also be the cause to determine nonresponsiveness (e.g., too high expectations of patients, the "honeymoon effect" [27]). Further information about secondary nonresponse and antibody development in other indication can be found in recent reviews [62, 63].

2.5. Development of antibody titer after termination of therapy

How the antibody titer developed after cessation of the Botulinum toxin therapy was analyzed in small clinical studies [64]. Thirteen patients treated for various distonic symptoms and with complete secondary treatment failure were analyzed overt time [64]. By applying the HDA to quantitate the titer of neutralizing antibodies in sera Dressler&Bigalke found that in 8/13 patients the titer decreased in the period between 500 and 1750 days. After between 1250 and 2250 days to such a low titer that complete therapy failure is unlikely as the authors assume. Five of the patient did not show decreasing antibody titer. The authors suggest that for some of the patients, botulinum toxin therapy could be reinitiated [64].

Hefter et al. analyzed the development of the antibody titer in a prospective, blinded cohort study including 37 patients with CD who had developed neutralizing antibodies and partial secondary nonresponse to prior therapy with ABO or ONA [65]. The patients received continuous treatment with INCO with 200 U and after 24 months with 300 U for up to 50 months. Ten patients (27%) in this study had a transient increase in titers of such antibodies in the first 24 months of treatment with INCO. However, for the majority of patients (84%), antibody titers declined to levels below the initial. At the end of the study, tests for neutralizing antibodies were either negative or below the lower detection limit in 23 patients (62%). The titer of 24 nonresponders not treated with INCO was also analyzed. Both cohorts, INCO treated and nontreated, showed a similar decline in antibody titer [65]. However, it is unclear whether the patients whose antibody titers decreased regained complete treatment benefit. In any case, the injection of INCO did not increase the antibody titer and one can assume that it was not recognized as an antigen in this long-term study because of the low protein load with this product.

3. Conclusions

The development of neutralizing antibodies in patients with CD or spasticity treated with botulinum toxin is rare. However, due to the large number of patients treated worldwide, it can be assumed that approximately 50,000 individuals become nonresponder. However, because the large difference in the sensitivity of the assays used it is not possible to assess the percentage of patients who will develop antibodies during the course of treatment. With respect of the high antigenic dose in the treatment with the BoNT/B product, neutralizing antibodies are detected much more frequently than with BoNT/A products. Whether the antibody titer is high enough to neutralize the injected dose of the neurotoxin might be different from patient to patient depending on the condition in the injected muscle, for example, how fast the neurotoxin molecules migrate to the motor endplate and escape from the antibody molecules, it might also depend on the distribution of the antibody molecules in the muscle tissue. Therefore, an antibody titer in a respective serum does not necessarily mean that the patient is unresponsive to botulinum toxin, and this is certainly a matter of the concentration of the antibodies in the muscle. The antibody concentration and the binding capacity of the antibodies to BoNT molecules determine whether the injected dose of the neurotoxin is only partly or completely neutralized. But if the immune system is already activated and a low titer is generated it can be assumed that further injections will increase the titer leading eventually to therapy failure. Unfortunately, systematic studies which analyze the development of low titers after further injections are missing.

Whether there are differences in the antigenic potential of botulinum toxin products which is not analyzed in head to head clinical studies and probably never will. All products containing complexing proteins generated antibody induced secondary nonresponse with various rates. There are no reports until now revealing that INCO induced secondary nonresponse in naïve patients. It can be assumed that the absence of other bacterial proteins and substances and a high specific potency of the product favor a low immunogenic potential. As already suggested since the beginning of botulinum toxin therapy, some obvious factors should be taken into account to avoid the formation of neutralizing antibodies: the dose should be as low as possible, just high enough to achieve the therapeutic effect and the injection should be as infrequent as possible. In the event that antibodies associated with nonresponsiveness are already present a different serotype could be applied. It has been shown that the antibody titer decreases over time; therefore, it could be advisable to monitor the antibody titer and reinitiate the therapy after the titer is low. This might take two or more years.

Author details

Jürgen Frevert[1] and Dirk Dressler[2*]

*Address all correspondence to: Dressler.Dirk@mh-hannover.de

1 Merz Pharmaceuticals GmbH, Potsdam, Germany

2 Medizinische Hochschule Hannover, Hannover, Germany

http://dx.doi.org/10.5772/64566

References

[1] Albanese A, Asmus F, Bhatia KP, Elia AE, Elibol B, Filippini G, Gasser T, Krauss JK, Nardocci N, Newton A, Valls-Solé: EFNS guidelines on diagnosis and treatment of primary dystonias. Eur J Neurol. 2011;18:5–18.

[2] Rossetto O, Pirazzini M, Montecucco C: Botulinum neurotoxins: genetic, structural and mechanistic insights. Nat Rev Microbiol. 2014;12:535–49.

[3] Montal M: Botulinum neurotoxin: a marvel of protein design. Annu Rev Biochem. 2010;79:591–617.

[4] Aoki KR, Guyer B: Botulinum toxin type A and other botulinum toxin serotypes: a comparative review of biochemical and pharmacological actions. Eur J Neurol. 2001;8(Suppl 5):21–9.

[5] Brunger AT, Rummel A: Receptor and substrate interactions of clostridial neurotoxins. Toxicon. 2009;54:550–60.

[6] Popoff MR, Poulain B: Bacterial toxins and the nervous system: neurotoxins and multipotential toxins interacting with neuronal cells. Toxins (Basel). 2010;2:683–737.

[7] Inoue K, Fujinaga Y, Watanabe T, et al: Molecular composition of *Clostridium botulinum* type A progenitor toxins. Infect Immun. 1996;64:1589–94.

[8] Inoue K, Fujinaga Y, Honke K, Arimitsu H, Mahmut N, Sakaguchi Y, Ohyama T, Watanabe T, Inoue K, Oguma K: *Clostridium botulinum* type A hemagglutinin-positive progenitor toxin (HA(+)-PTX) binds to oligosaccharides containing Gal beta1–4GlcNAc through one subcomponent of haemagglutinin (HA1). Microbiology. 2001;(Pt 4):811–9.

[9] Purcell RT, Lockey RF: Immunologic responses to therapeutic biologic agents. J Investig Allergol Clin Immunol. 2008;18(5):335–42.

[10] Critchfield J: Considering the immune response to botulinum toxin. Clin J Pain. 2002;18(6 Suppl):S133–41.

[11] Dressler D, Hallett M: Immunological aspects of Botox, Dysport and Myobloc/NeuroBloc. Eur J Neurol. 2006;13(Suppl 1):11–5.

[12] Dressler D: Clinical features of antibody-induced complete secondary failure of botulinum toxin therapy. Eur Neurol. 2002;48:26–9.

[13] Dolimbek BZ, Aoki KR, Steward LE, Jankovic J, Atassi MZ: Mapping of the regions on the heavy chain of botulinum neurotoxin A (BoNT/A) recognized by antibodies of cervical dystonia patients with immunoresistance to BoNT/A. Mol Immunol. 2007;44:1029–41.

[14] Atassi MZ, Dolimbek BZ: Mapping of the antibody-binding regions on the HN-domain (residues 449–859) of botulinum neurotoxin A with antitoxin antibodies from four host

species. Full profile of the continuous antigenic regions of the H-chain of botulinum neurotoxin A. Protein J. 2004;23:39–52.

[15] Jankovic J, Schwartz K: Response and immunoresistance to botulinum toxin injections. Neurology. 1995;45:1743–6.

[16] Jankovic J, Schwartz KS: Clinical correlates of response to botulinum toxin injections. Arch Neurol. 1991;48:1253–1256.

[17] Greene P, Fahn S, Diamond B: Development of resistance to botulinum toxin type A in patients with torticollis. Mov Disord. 1994;9(2):213–7.

[18] Jankovic J, Vuong KD, Ahsan J: Comparison of efficacy and immunogenicity of original versus current botulinum toxin in cervical dystonia. Neurology. 2003;60:1186–8.

[19] Göschel H, Wohlfarth K, Frevert J, Dengler R, Bigalke H: Botulinum A toxin therapy: neutralizing and nonneutralizing antibodies—therapeutic consequences. Exp Neurol. 1997;147:96–102.

[20] Wang L, Sun Y, Yang W, Lindo P, Singh BR.: Type A botulinum neurotoxin complex proteins differentially modulate host response of neuronal cells. Toxicon. 2014;82:52–60.

[21] Iwasaki A, Medzhitov R: Regulation of adaptive immunity by the innate immune system. Science. 2010;327:291–5.

[22] Sharon N, Lis H: History of lectins: from hemagglutinins to biological recognition molecules. Glycobiology. 2004;14:53R–62R.

[23] Hatheway CL, Dang C (1994): Immunogenicity of the neurotoxins of *Clostridium botulinum*. In: Jankovic J, Hallett M (eds). Therapy with botulinum toxin. Marcel Dekker, New York, pp. 93–107.

[24] Shone C, Wilton-Smith P, Appleton N, Hambleton P, Modi N, Gatley S, Melling J: Monoclonal antibody-based immunoassay for type A *Clostridium botulinum* toxin is comparable to he mouse bioassay. Appl Environ Microbiol. 1985;50:63–7.

[25] Hanna PA, Jankovic J: Mouse bioassay versus Western blot assay for botulinum toxin antibodies: correlation with clinical response. Neurology. 1998;50:1624–1629.

[26] Dressler D, Dirnberger G: Botulinum toxin antibody testing: comparison between the immunoprecipitation assay and the mouse diaphragm assay. Eur Neurol. 2001;45:257–60.

[27] Lange O, Bigalke H, Dengler R, Wegner F, deGroot M, Wohlfarth K: Neutralizing antibodies and secondary therapy failure after treatment with botulinum toxin type A: much ado about nothing?. Clin Neuropharmacol. 2009:32:213–218.

[28] Kessler KR, Benecke R: The EBD test—a clinical test for the detection of antibodies to botulinum toxin type A. Mov Disord. 1997;12:95–99.

http://dx.doi.org/10.5772/64566

[29] Brin MF, Comella CL, Jankovic J, Lai F, Naumann M; CD-017 BoNTA Study Group.: Long-term treatment with botulinum toxin type A in cervical dystonia has low immunogenicity by mouse protectionassay. Mov Disord. 2008;23:1353–60.

[30] Dressler D, Bigalke H, Rothwell JC: The sternocleidomastoid test: an in vivo assay to investigate botulinum toxin antibody formation in humans. J Neurol. 2000;247:630–2.

[31] Birklein F, Erbguth F: Sudomotor testing discriminates between subjects with and without antibodies against botulinum. Mov Disord. 2000;15(1):146–9.

[32] European Medicines Agency (EMA): Guideline on immunogenicity assessment of biotechnology-derived therapeutic proteins [online]. Available from URL: www.ema.europa.eu/pdfs/human/biosimilar/1432706en.pdf.

[33] Herrmann J, Geth K, Mall V, Bigalke H, Schulte Mönting J, Linder M, Kirschner J, Berweck S, Korinthenberg R, Heinen F, Fietzek UM: Clinical impact of antibody formation to botulinum toxin A in children. Ann Neurol. 2004;55(5):732–5.

[34] Naumann M, Carruthers A, Carruthers J, Aurora SK, Zafonte R, Abu-Shakra S, Boodhoo T, Miller-Messana MA, Demos G, James L, Beddingfield F, VanDenburgh A, Chapman MA, Brin MF: Meta-analysis of neutralizing antibody conversion with onabotulinumtoxinA (BOTOX) across multiple indications. Mov Disord. 2010:25:2211–2218.

[35] Mejia NI, Vuong KD, Jankovic J: Long-term botulinum toxin efficacy, safety, and immunogenicity. Mov Disord. 2005;20:592–7.

[36] Frevert J: Content of botulinum neurotoxin in Botox/Vistabel, Dysport/ Azzalure, and Xeomin/Bocouture: Drugs R D. 2010;10:67–73.

[37] Callaway JE, Arezzo JC, Grethlein AJ: Botulinum toxin type B: an overview of its biochemistry and preclinical pharmacology. Semin Cutan Med Surg. 2001;20(2):127–36.

[38] Jankovic J, Hunter C, Dolimbek BZ, Dolimbek GS, Adler CH, Brashear A, Comella CL, Gordon M, Riley DE, Sethi K, Singer C, Stacy M, Tarsy D, Atassi MZ: Clinico-immunologic aspects of botulinum toxin type B treatment of cervical dystonia. Neurology. 2006;67:2233–2235.

[39] Dressler D, Dimberger G: Botulinum toxin therapy: risk factors for therapy failure [abstract]: Mov Disord. 2000;15(Suppl 2):51.

[40] Evidente VG, Truong D, Jankovic J, Comella CL, Grafe, Hanschmann A: IncobotulinumtoxinA (Xeomin") injected for blepharospasm or cervical dystonia according to patient needs is well tolerated. J Neurol Sci. 2014;346(1–2):116–20.

[41] Fabbri M, Leodori G, Fernandes RM, Bhidayasiri R, Marti MJ, Colosimo C, Ferreira JJ: Neutralizing antibody and botulinum toxin therapy: a systematic review and meta-analysis. Neurotox Res. 2015, 29(1):105-117.

[42] Brin MF, Comella CL, Jankovic J, Lai F, Naumann M: Longterm treatment with botulinum toxin type A in cervical dystonia has low immunogenicity by mouse protection assay. Mov Disord. 2008;23:1353–1360.

[43] Truong D, Brodsky M, Lew M, Brashear A, Jankovic J, Molho E, Orlova O, Timerbaeva S: Long-term efficacy and safety of botulinum toxin type A (Dysport) in cervical dystonia. Parkinsonism. Relat Disord. 2010;16:316–323.

[44] Coleman C, Hubble J, Schwab J, Beffy JL, Picaut P, Morte C.Immunoresistance in cervical dystonia patients after treatment with abobotulinumtoxinA.Int J Neurosci. 2012: 358–62.

[45] Kessler KR, Skutta M, Benecke R Long-term treatment of cervical dystonia with botulinum toxin A: efficacy, safety, and antibody frequency. German Dystonia Study Group. J Neurol. 1999; 246:265–274.

[46] Haussermann P, Marczoch S, Klinger C, Landgrebe M, Conrad B, Ceballos-Baumann A (2004) Long-term follow-up of cervical dystonia patients treated with botulinum toxin A: Mov Disord 19:303–308.

[47] Comella CL, Jankovic J, Truong DD, Hanschmann A, Grafe S: U.S. XEOMIN Cervical Dystonia Study Group. Efficacy and safety of incobotulinumtoxinA (NT 201, XEO-MIN®, botulinum neurotoxin type A, without accessory proteins) in patients with cervical dystonia. J Neurol Sci. 2011;308(1–2):103–109.

[48] Evidente VG, Fernandez HH, LeDoux MS, MS, Brashear A, Grafe S, Hanschmann A, Comella CL: A randomized, double-blind study of repeated incobotulinumtoxinA (Xeomin(®)) in cervical dystonia: J Neural Transm. 2013;120(12):1699–1707.

[49] Sethi KD, Rodriguez R, Olayinka B: Satisfaction with botulinum toxin treatment: a cross-sectional survey of patients with cervical dystonia. J Med Econ. 2012;15(3):419–423.

[50] Fernandez HH, Pappert EJ, Comella CL, Evidente VG, Truong DD, Verma A, Jankovic J.: Efficacy and safety of incobotulinumtoxinA in subjects previously treated with botulinum toxin versus toxin-naïve subjects with cervical dystonia: Tremor Other Hyerkinet Mov (N Y). 2013;3.

[51] Benecke R: Xeomin in the treatment of cervical dystonia. Eur J Neurol. 2009;16(Suppl 2):6–10.

[52] Dressler D, Paus S, Seitzinger A, Gebhardt B, Kupsch A: Long-term efficacy and safety of incobotulinumtoxinA injections in patients with cervical dystonia. J Neurol Neurosurg Psychiatry. 2013;84(9):1014–1019.

[53] Chinnapongse RB, Lew MF, Ferreira JJ, Gullo KL, Nemeth PR, Zhang Y. Cl: Immunogenicity and long-term efficacy of botulinum toxin type B in the treatment of cervical dystonia: report of 4 prospective, multicenter trials. Clin Neuropharmacol. 2012;35(5): 215–23.

[54] Dressler D, Bigalke H: Botulinum toxin type B de novo therapy of cervical dystonia: frequency of antibody induced therapy failure. J Neurol. 2005;252:904–907.

[55] Yablon SA, Brashear A, Gordon MF, Elovic EP, Turkel CC, Daggett S, Liu J, Brin MF: Formation of neutralizing antibodies in patients receiving botulinum toxin type A for treatment of poststroke spasticity: a pooled-data analysis of three clinical trials. Clin Ther. 2007;29:683–690.

[56] Elovic EP, Brashear A, Kaelin D, Liu J, Millis SR, Barron R, Turkel C: Repeated treatments with botulinum toxin type a produce sustained decreases in the limitations associated with focal upper-limb poststroke spasticity for caregivers and patients. Arch Phys Med Rehabil. 2008;89:799–806.

[57] Bakheit AM, Fedorova NV, Skoromets AA, Timerbaeva SL, Bhakta BB, Coxon L: The beneficial antispasticity effect of botulinum toxin type A is maintained after repeated treatment cycles. J Neurol Neurosurg Psychiatry. 2004;75:1558–1561.

[58] Kanovsky P, Slawek J, Denes Z, Platz T, Sassin I, Comes G, Grafe S: Efficacy and safety of botulinum neurotoxin NT 201 in poststroke upper limb spasticity. Clin Neuropharmacol. 2009;32:259.

[59] Dressler D, Rychlik R, Kreimendahl F, Schnur N, Lambert-Baumann J: Long-term efficacy and safety of incobotulinumtoxinA and conventional treatment of poststroke arm spasticity: a prospective, non-interventional, open-label, parallel-group study. BMJ Open. 2015;5(12).

[60] Brashear A, McAfee AL, Kuhn ER, Fyffe J: Botulinum toxin type B in upper-limb poststroke spasticity: a double-blind, placebo-controlled trial. Arch Phys Med Rehabil. 2004;85:705–709.

[61] Dressler D, Bigalke H, Benecke R: Botulinum toxin type B in antibody-induced botulinum toxin type A therapy failure. J Neurol. 2003;250:967–969.

[62] Naumann M, Boo LM, Ackerman AH, Gallagher CJ: Immunogenicity of botulinum toxins. J Neural Transm (Vienna). 2013;120(2):275–90.

[63] Benecke R: Clinical relevance of botulinum toxin:immunogenicity. BioDrugs. 2012;26(2):1–9.

[64] Dressler D, Bigalke H: Botulinum toxin antibody type A titres after cessation of botulinum toxin therapy. Mov Disord. 2002;17(1):170–3.

[65] Hefter H, Hartmann C, Kahlen U, Moll M, Bigalke H: Prospective analysis of neutralising antibody titres in secondary non-responders under continuous treatment with a botulinumtoxin type A preparation free of complexing proteins – a single cohort 4-year follow-up study. BMJ Open. 2012;2(4).

Section 3

Botulinum Toxin Therapy: Applied in Dystonia and Spasticity

Chapter 5

What Practical Tips Can I Suggest during Botulinum Toxin Injection?

Woong-Woo Lee and Beomseok Jeon

Additional information is available at the end of the chapter

http://dx.doi.org/10.5772/64144

Abstract

Botulinum toxin injections are effective for hyperactivities of muscles and glands that are mediated by acetylcholine (Ach) release in neuronal terminal. The effects of botulinum toxin are reversible because the involved nerves build new sprouts and synapses with time. Thus, botulinum toxin is relatively safe and repeated applications are needed. To maximize effects of botulinum toxin without side effects, understanding the action mechanism of botulinum toxin and determining appropriate target sites are very important. Many guidelines have already been published and provided useful information for these. Therefore, in this chapter, we concentrate more on practical tips for botulinum toxin injections.

Keywords: botulinum toxin, acetylcholine, dystonia, spasticity, hemifacial spasm

1. Introduction

The natural Botulinum neurotoxin (BoNT) is produced by *Clostridium botulinum*, a type of spore-producing gram-positive bacilli. Sources of botulism poisoning are soil, honey, canned foods, etc., because *C. botulinum* thrives in anaerobic conditions. BoNT can be denatured at over 80°C (176°F). BoNT consists of a heavy chain and light chain, which are polypeptides linked by a disulfide bond [1]. Initially, the heavy chain binds to the surface of a nerve cell. The light chain, which acts as a Zn-dependent protease, is internalized into the nerve cell, and then, it cleaves specific soluble N-ethylmaleimide sensitive factor attachment protein receptor (SNARE) proteins: synaptosome-associated protein (SNAP-25), syntaxin, and vesicle-associated membrane protein (VAMP). There are several serotypes of BoNT. Type A, C1, and E break down SNAP-25; type C hydrolyzes syntaxin, and type B, D, F, and G block the function of

VAMP. As a result, acetylcholine (Ach) remains inside the vesicles and cannot be released into the synaptic cleft. The duration of the BoNT activity is generally limited to several weeks or several months because the involved nerves form new sprouts and synapses that can release Ach [2].

The first agent, which was approved by the Food and Drug Administration in 1989, is Botox® (Allergan Inc, Irvine, CA, USA). Botulinum toxin type A (BoNT/A) is most commonly used these days: Botox®, OnabotulinumtoxinA; Dysport®, AbobotulinumtoxinA; Xeomin®, IncobotulinumtoxinA; Hengli/CBTX-A®, Chinese botulinumtoxin A; Neuronox/Meditoxin®, South Korea botulinumtoxin A, etc. Botulinum toxin type B is also frequently used: Myobloc®/Neurobloc®, RimabotulinumtoxinB.

The practitioners of BoNT injection need to remember that BoNT is a protein. This means that BoNT can denature easily and contribute to the generation of neutralizing antibodies. BoNT has to be stored at 2–8 °C (36–46 °F) and administrated only for a limited time [3–5]. Freezing, light exposure, and shaking should be avoided. To reduce the incidence of antibody generation, the following are recommended: maintain at least a 3-month interval between injections; use the smallest possible dose, and avoid booster injections. Detailed prescription information for widely used BoNTs is summarized in **Table 1** [3–5].

	Botox® [3]	**Dysport® [4]**	**Myobloc® [5]**
Contents	OnabotulinumtoxinA	AbobotulinumtoxinA	RimabotulinumtoxinB
	Human albumin	Human albumin	Human albumin
	Sodium chloride	Lactose	Sodium succinate
		Cow's milk proteins	Sodium chloride
Target SNARE protein	SNAP-25	SNAP-25	VAMP
Storage	Store at 2–8°C (36–46°F)	Store at 2–8°C (36–46 °F)	Store at 2–8°C (36–46°F)
	Inject BoNT within 24 hours	Inject BoNT within 24 hours	Inject BoNT within 4 hours, once diluted
		Do not freeze	Do not freeze
		Protect from light	Do not shake
			Protect from light
Reconstitution	Sterile, preservative-free 0.9% sodium chloride		Provided as solution (pH 5.6)
			Can be diluted with normal saline
Indications and usage	Cervical dystonia	Cervical dystonia	Cervical dystonia
	Blepharospasm	Glabella lines	
	Spasticity in adult	Upper limb spasticity in adult	

http://dx.doi.org/10.5772/64144

	Botox® [3]	Dysport® [4]	Myobloc® [5]
	Chronic migraine		
	Strabismus		
	Axillary hyperhidrosis		
	Overactive bladder		
Contraindications	Hypersensitivity to any BoNT	Hypersensitivity to any BoNT	Hypersensitivity to any BoNT
	Infection	Infection	Infection
		Allergy to cow's milk protein	
Limit of a total dose	400 Units	1000 Units	NA
Minimal interval	3 months	12 weeks	NA
Side effects	Generalized weakness, diplopia, ptosis, dysphagia, dysphonia, dysarthria, urinary incontinence, breathing difficulties		
	Pain, inflammation, bleeding		
	Flu, rhinitis, pharyngitis		
Drug interactions	Aminoglycosides and other agents interfering with neuromuscular transmission (eg. Curare-like agents)		
	Anticholinergics		
	Muscle relaxants		
	Other BoNT		
Cautions	Pregnancy (Category C)		
	Nursing mothers		
	Pediatric/geriatric use		
Immunogenicity	Positive antibodies: 0.0–1.2%	Positive antibodies: 0.0–3.6%	Neutralizing activity
	Risk factors: frequent intervals, higher doses		- 1 years: 10% (for 36% ELISA-positive cases)
			- 18 months: 18% (for 50% ELISA-positive cases)

SNARE, soluble N-ethlymaleimide sensitive factor attachment protein receptor; SNAP-25, synaptosome-associated protein; VAMP, vesicle-associated membrane protein; BoNT, botulinum neurotoxin; NA, not applicable.
*The incidence of antibodies are highly dependent on the methodology of the assay. Therefore, the simple comparisons between different BoNTs are illogical.

Table 1. Summary of prescribing information.

Early BoNTs did not overcome the following problems: short-lasting effects, necrotizing problem, and systematic toxicity [6]. However, there have been remarkable advances since Scott et al. [7] successfully improved strabismus with purified BoNT injections. Now BoNT is widely used to reduce the hyperactivity of muscles or glands mediated by Ach release [1]. For neurological disorders, BoNT can be effectively used for hyperkinetic movement disorders (dystonia, hemifacial spasm, myoclonus, myokymia, tremor, etc.), spasticity, drooling, and chronic migraines. Applications for strabismus, spasms of the gastrointestinal tract or genito-urinary tract, and cosmetic work are possible.

In this chapter, although there have been many guidelines published, we focus more on the practical tips for BoNT injections in the treatment of several neurological symptoms.

2. Before botulinum toxin injection

2.1. Selection of appropriate patients for botulinum toxin injections

The principle action mechanism of BoNT is to block the release of Ach from presynaptic nerve terminals. Therefore, the Ach-mediated hyperactivities of muscles and glands could be good targets for BoNT therapy. The following list shows representative indications for BoNT injection.

- Hyperkinetic movement disorders

  o Dystonia (cervical dystonia, blepharospasm, oro-mandibular dystonia, limb dystonia, laryngeal dystonia, etc.)

  o Hemifacial spasm

  o Myoclonus, myokymia, tremor, dyskinesia, tics, etc.

- Other neurological disorders

  o Spasticity

  o Headache (chronic tension type headache, chronic migraine)

  o Drooling, etc.

- Other disorders

  o Strabismus

  o Hyperhidrosis

  o Spasm or spasticity of the gastro-intestinal and genito-urinary tracts

  o Cosmestic applications, etc.

The cautions and contraindications are as important as the proper indications. Patients with neurological disorders involving anterior horn cells, peripheral nerves, neuro-muscular junctions, and muscles require special care when injecting BoNT. Concomitant use of drugs, which could affect neuro-muscular transmission or cause muscle weakness, is also not recommended (**Table 1**) [3–5]. In addition, most BoNTs do not guarantee the safety of pregnant women, nursing mothers, and pediatric patients. Hypersensitivities to any of the BoNTs or their components and the infection of target sites are important contraindications. Especially, Dysport® is contraindicated in patients with allergies to cow's milk protein [4]. Anti-platelet or anti-coagulation agents could cause a hematoma.

2.2. Selection of botulinum toxin

Despite past studies using different types of BoNT, it is unclear which one is the most effective BoNT. Furthermore, it is generally accepted that the doses between different BoNT products are not interchangeable [3–5, 8–10]. However, in real practice, patients who have been treated with different BoNT products could visit your clinic any time. In this regard, a simple conversion ratio between Botox® and Dysport® was made [11]. Based on the average recommended dose of Dysport®(500 Units) and Botox® (200 Units) for patients with cervical dystonia, a conversion ratio of 2.5:1 was assumed and it was found that Dysport® showed no inferiority to Botox® at this ratio. The ratio of 2.5:1 has the practical advantage by simplifying the interchanging process. This issue will be addressed in detail later.

3. Preparing botulinum toxin injection

3.1. Reconstitution

The widely used solvent for reconstituting BoNT is 0.9% normal saline. Hypotonic saline or distilled water is not suitable as a solvent because it could cause pain. Recently one preliminary study suggested that reconstituting BoNT with Ringer acetate could reduce the injection site pain rather than with normal saline by normalizing the pH values of the solution [12]. Myobloc® is provided as a solution (pH 5.6) that can be used as is or diluted with normal saline [5].

Regardless of the BoNT subtype, one unit of BoNT was defined as the calculated median intraperitoneal lethal dose (LD_{50}) in mice. However, the biological activity varies between BoNTs. Although there is no consensus for the conversion ratio, we use the ratio of 2.5:1 for Dysport® and Botox® because the non-inferiority of Dysport® has already been proven [11]. On the assumption that the ratio of 2.5:1 is bioequivalent, the practitioner can make two kinds of solutions (**Table 2**). To make a solution with a high concentration, 1 ml of 0.9% normal saline is needed for 1 ample (100 Units) of Botox® and 2 ml of 0.9% normal saline for 1 ample (500 Units) of Dysport®. For a solution with a low concentration, 2 ml and 4 ml are mixed with 1 ample of Botox® and Dysport®, respectively. Then, the same volume of each solution indicates the same potency (**Table 2**). It means that physicians do not need complicated calculations. Because the same conversion ratio (2.5:1) is also applied to the limitations for the total doses of Dysport® (1000 Units) and Botox® (400 Units), we believe that it is very simple and practical.

After injecting normal saline for reconstitution, the next step is to mix gently to minimize unnecessary destruction of the toxin. Because the available time is short after reconstitution (within 24 hours for Botox® and Dysport®) [3, 4], it is more efficient to inject BoNT after gathering sufficient numbers of patients who need BoNT treatment.

	Botox®, OnabotulinumtoxinA	Dysport®, AbobotulinumtoxinA
Units per 1 ample	100 Units	500 Units
Method #1 (high concentration)	100 Units (1 ample): 1 ml of 0.9% N/S	500 Units (1 ample): 2 ml of 0.9% N/S
	→ 0.1 ml solution = 10 Units of Ona-BoNT/A	→ 0.1 ml solution = 25 Units of Abo-BoNT/A
	→ 0.01 ml solution = 1 Unit of Ona-BoNT/A	→ 0.01 ml solution = 2.5 Units of Abo-BoNT/A
Method #2 (low concentration)	100 Units (1 ample): 2 ml of 0.9% N/S	500 Units (1 ample): 4 ml of 0.9% N/S
	→ 0.1 ml solution = 5 Units of Ona-BoNT/A	→ 0.1 ml solution = 12.5 Units of Abo-BoNT/A
	→ 0.01 ml solution = 0.5 Units of Ona-BoNT/A	→ 0.01 ml solution = 1.25 Units of Abo-BoNT/A

BoNT/A, botulinum neurotoxin type A.

Table 2. Practical tips of conversion between Botox® and Dysport®.

3.2. Preparation of the syringe and needle

Generally, a 1-ml syringe, which can control the volume by 0.01 ml, is preferred. The practitioner needs 0.03–0.05 ml more volume than the target volume, taking into consideration the dead space inside of the needle. After the syringe is filled properly with the BoNT solution, the practitioner should remove the air. The following are tips for removing air bubbles and aligning the needle.

- Draw down the syringe quickly while holding the cap of syringe. It is based on the inertia effect, and just one time is enough to collect bubbles on top. Tapping the body is also available.
- Pull slightly back, before pushing forward, the plunger of the syringe. It will be helpful in saving the BoNT in the dead space of the needle.
- Rotate the bevel of the needle in the same direction with the scale marks of the syringe.

The selection of the injection needle depends on the target sites. Because most facial muscles are thin and close to the skin, a thin and short needle such as a 23- or 24-gauge needle is suitable for the delivery of BoNT solution. In contrast, neck and limb muscles are thick, large, and located relatively deep from skin. Thus, a thick and long needle such as a 21-gauge needle is necessary.

http://dx.doi.org/10.5772/64144

4. Injecting botulinum toxin

4.1. Determining target sites

BoNT injection is recommended for use in only limited areas. The reasons for the limited use are because of the total dose and cost of BoNT. Therefore, determining the target is the most important procedure in treatment with BoNT.

Determining target sites has the same meaning as finding symptomatic muscles. It is not difficult to locate target sites for disorders with static muscular hypertonia (such as fixed dystonia or spasticity). However, mobile hyperkinetic movement disorders are another matter. Especially for mobile dystonia, finding target muscles is not simple because the direction of abnormal movement seems to be irregular or changes every moment. Ultrasonography, computed tomography, magnetic resonance imaging, and electromyography (EMG) are supportive tools to help ascertain the target [13]. In particular, EMG can provide dynamic information and help in the precise injection of BoNT to target muscles in real time. However it should be kept in mind that EMG is not a substitute for knowledge of anatomy and is a mere supportive tool. Another important thing is to avoid BoNT injections near sites where side effects occur frequently. Particularly the procedure for head and neck requires special care.

Practical tips for examining patients and determining target sites are introduced below.

4.1.1. Cervical dystonia

The final posture of cervical dystonia (CD) patients consists of a combination of dystonic muscle contractions, compensatory movements, and secondary musculo-skeletal changes. Therefore, examination in various situations is helpful in differentiating target dystonic muscles from the others.

Before the examination, enough exposure of the neck and adjacent muscles is very important. This procedure is essential for precise inspection. In addition, sensory trick by scarf or clothes could be eliminated. Then, the physicians should see the rotation and deviation of neck and adjacent muscles on a neutral position, and describe how they are seen. It can be summarized as the combination of turning to one side (torticollis), tilting or shifting to one side (laterocollis), bending forward (antecollis) or backward (retrocollis). Shoulder elevation is frequently accompanied.

Here are several methods to distinguish compensatory movements. The physicians have to tell the patients "let the neck and shoulder relax as they move", and make them walk repeatedly. Palpation of the candidate muscles is helpful in assessing whether they are hypertrophic or contain bands. The features of dystonia such as task-specificity, overflow, and null-point could also be important clues. Especially for tremulous CD, if a tremor diminishes at a specific position, the muscles inducing that position would be affected by dystonia. Short-term follow-up can reveal critical information. The effect of BoNT for CD is generally maximized within 2 or 3 weeks after injection. Therefore, early visits can provide information whether previous target sites were appropriate as well as whether the patient is a BoNT non-responder. The dynamic progression of dystonia is another reason why follow-up is important.

4.1.2. Facial involuntary movements

Determining target sites in facial involuntary movements is relatively simple compared to CD. Therefore, when BoNT is injected into the face, avoiding side effects is given much weight. The face contains other important anatomical structures such as the eye balls, lacrimal ducts, salivary glands, nerves, and vessels. The direction of the needle always must head away from the eye balls. Two canaliculi per eye exist in the medial canthus. BoNT injection into the lower canaliculus generally is avoided because it is believed to have a main role in transporting tears to the lacrimal sac and nasolacrimal duct. When injecting into the masseter muscle, it is better to preserve the lower posterior portion where the parotid gland is placed.

Asymmetry and ptosis should be considered. To prevent asymmetry, injections are often given also on the contralateral side. To prevent ptosis, BoNT injections to the mid-portions of the upper eyelid and frontalis area are avoided. Especially, when the orbicularis oculi is the target, injection into the pretarsal area has stronger effects and less frequent ptosis than injections into the preseptal area [14, 15].

4.1.3. Limb dystonia

Using overflow phenomenon and mirror movement is a good way to differentiate main symptomatic spasms from compensatory ones [16]. If hand dystonia is too complex to determine a target, an EMG-guided approach will be useful. However, it is not easy to inject only into the real target site because the hands are comprised of small muscles for delicate movements. And paralysis of specific muscle rather can cause great inconvenience in most situations except when that specific task is performed.

4.2. Determining target volume

Once the target muscles for BoNT injection have been chosen, the next step is determining how much BoNT and how many injection sites are required. The recommended volumes for several target muscles are provided in the prescription information [3–5]. However, the response varies from person to person and information for every possible indication is not included. Thus, the injection volume and site should be individualized taking into consideration race, sex, age, medical condition, etc.

The followings are additional helpful tips in determining the injection volume.

- For larger target muscles, a larger volume of BoNT is required.
- It is safer to apply a low dose first.
- Imagining the diffusion pattern of BoNT is important.

Borodic et al. [17] reported several important features for the BoNT/A diffusion pattern in the longissimus dorsi of rabbits: the diffusion of BoNT/A occurred in a dose-dependent manner;

the spread pattern in the injected muscle was more linear than in a remote muscle of the same distance; lower doses did not affect a different muscle located 45 mm from the injection site while higher doses diffused even into that muscle. This study supports the concept that injection into multiple sites with lower doses could reduce side effects by preventing the diffusion of BoNT, in other words its biological effect, to other muscles beyond the injection site [18]. Therefore, Rosales et al. [19] recommended a "high potency, low dilution" of BoNT/A for oromandibular, lingual, cranial, cervical, and distal limb dystonias, which are small and localized targets. In contrast, A "low potency, high dilution" of BoNT/A is more useful for big muscles.

4.3. Methods of botulinum toxin injection

The method of injection mainly depends on the anatomical features of target sites.

Superficial fat compartments are distributed throughout the entire face excluding the upper eyelids, nose, and mouth [20]. Most facial muscles are located just beneath the skin and subcutaneous fat, whereas peri-ocular and peri-oral areas have little fatty tissue. Facial skin is relatively thin compared to the other parts. Especially, the skin thickness of the palpebral areas is only around 0.5 mm. Therefore, when the orbicularis oculi or orbicularis oris muscle is the target, the needle should be inserted horizontally to skin as much as possible although more pain at the injection site is inevitable. Smoothing out skin wrinkles is important for easy needling. Vesicle formation is also recommended in these areas because it seems to be helpful in localizing the extent of chemo-denervation. For other facial muscles, the angle between needle and skin needs to be set a little bit higher so that the needle can be inserted into a deeper location. Another important consideration in facial muscle anatomy is that the facial muscles have few muscle spindles except in jaw muscles. It refers that BoNT injections directly impact on extrafusal muscle fibers in face.

On the other hand, neck and limb muscles are large and located more deeply. For effective delivery of BoNT, a long needle inserted perpendicularly to the skin is necessary. This direction of insertion is also good for reducing pain. Grasping and fixing muscles are essential for precise targeting. Postures of activating relevant muscles and imaging- or EMG-guided methods may be of great help to approach deep muscles. Before administering the BoNT solution, pulling back is required to ascertain whether the needle reaches the target muscle or adjunctive vessel.

5. Conclusion

To provide the appropriate BoNT treatment, the practitioner should be well informed of the etio-pathogenesis of disorders and the anatomy of the target area, as well as the action mechanism of BoNT and methods of storage and injection. Patients must also understand that BoNT treatment is just a way to relieve symptoms, and not treatment for underlying causes. Repeated applications of BoNT are required because the effects last for 3 months on average. Paradoxically, BoNT is a reversible and very safe toxin in terms of side effects. We hope that the guides of this chapter are very helpful in understanding and using BoNT in a clinical setting.

Author details

Woong-Woo Lee[1] and Beomseok Jeon[2*]

*Address all correspondence to: brain@snu.ac.kr

1 Department of Neurology, Eulji General Hospital, Seoul, Korea

2 Department of Neurology, Seoul National University Hospital, Seoul, Korea

References

[1] Jankovic J. Botulinum toxin in clinical practice. Journal of Neurology, Neurosurgery, and Psychiatry. 2004;75(7):951-7.

[2] Rosales RL, Bigalke H, Dressler D. Pharmacology of botulinum toxin: differences between type A preparations. European Journal of Neurology. 2006;13(Suppl 1):2-10.

[3] Allergan. Botox prescribing information [Internet]. 2016. Available from: http://www.allergan.com/assets/pdf/botox_pi.pdf [Accessed: 2016-03-14]

[4] Ipsen. Dysport prescribing information [Internet]. 2012. Available from: http://www.dysport.com/hcp/PDFs/Dysport_Patiens_PI_Aug2012.pdf [Accessed: 2016-03-14]

[5] Solstice Neurosciences. Myobloc prescribing information [Internet]. 2010. Available from: http://www.myobloc.com/hp_about/PI_5-19-10.pdf [Accessed: 2016-03-14]

[6] Scott AB, Rosenbaum A, Collins CC. Pharmacologic weakening of extraocular muscles. Investigative Ophthalmology. 1973;12(12):924-7.

[7] Scott AB. Botulinum toxin injection into extraocular muscles as an alternative to strabismus surgery. Ophthalmology. 1980;87(10):1044-9.

[8] Ravenni R, De Grandis D, Mazza A. Conversion ratio between Dysport and Botox in clinical practice: an overview of available evidence. Neurological Sciences. 2013;34(7):1043-8.

[9] Rystedt A, Nyholm D, Naver H. Clinical experience of dose conversion ratios between 2 botulinum toxin products in the treatment of cervical dystonia. Clinical Neuropharmacology. 2012;35(6):278-82.

[10] Bihari K. Safety, effectiveness, and duration of effect of BOTOX after switching from Dysport for blepharospasm, cervical dystonia, and hemifacial spasm dystonia, and hemifacial spasm. Current Medical Research and Opinion. 2005;21(3):433-8.

[11] Yun JY, Kim JW, Kim HT, Chung SJ, Kim JM, Cho JW, et al. Dysport and Botox at a ratio of 2.5:1 units in cervical dystonia: a double-blind, randomized study. Movement Disorders. 2015;30(2):206-13.

[12] Dressler D, Saberi FA, Bigalke H. Botulinum neurotoxin therapy: reduction of injection site pain by pH normalization. Toxicon. 2015;93:S20-S21.

[13] Grigoriu AI, Dinomais M, Remy-Neris O, Brochard S. Impact of injection-guiding techniques on the effectiveness of botulinum toxin for the treatment of focal spasticity and dystonia: a systematic review. Archives of Physical Medicine and Rehabilitation. 2015;96(11):2067-78.

[14] Albanese A, Bentivoglio AR, Colosimo C, Galardi G, Maderna L, Tonali P. Pretarsal injections of botulinum toxin improve blepharospasm in previously unresponsive patients. Journal of Neurology, Neurosurgery, and Psychiatry. 1996;60(6):693-4.

[15] Cakmur R, Ozturk V, Uzunel F, Donmez B, Idiman F. Comparison of preseptal and pretarsal injections of botulinum toxin in the treatment of blepharospasm and hemifacial spasm. Journal of Neurology. 2002;249(1):64-8.

[16] Karp BI. Botulinum toxin physiology in focal hand and cranial dystonia. Toxins (Basel). 2012;4(11):1404-14.

[17] Borodic GE, Ferrante R, Pearce LB, Smith K. Histologic assessment of dose-related diffusion and muscle fiber response after therapeutic botulinum A toxin injections. Movement Disorders. 1994;9(1):31-9.

[18] Blackie JD, Lees AJ. Botulinum toxin treatment in spasmodic torticollis. Journal of Neurology, Neurosurgery, and Psychiatry. 1990;53(8):640-3.

[19] Rosales RL, Ng AR, Santos MM, Fernandez HH. The broadening application of chemodenervation in X-linked dystonia-parkinsonism (Part II): an open-label experience with botulinum toxin-A (Dysport(R)) injections for oromandibular, lingual, and truncal-axial dystonias. The International Journal of Neuroscience. 2011;121(Suppl 1): 44-56.

[20] Rohrich RJ, Pessa JE. The fat compartments of the face: anatomy and clinical implications for cosmetic surgery. Plastic and Reconstructive Surgery. 2007;119(7):2219-27.

Chapter 6

How Effective and Safe is Botulinum Toxin Therapy in Cervical Dystonia: The Current Stand

Roland Dominic G. Jamora and Anthony N. Piano

Additional information is available at the end of the chapter

http://dx.doi.org/10.5772/64717

Abstract

Cervical dystonia (CD) is the most common focal dystonia that is characterized by involuntary contraction of cervical muscles causing abnormal head movements and postures. The treatment for CD was previously limited to oral medications, however, with consequent systemic side effects. In recent years, botulinum toxin (BoNT) has demonstrated efficacy in several studies and thus has received level A recommendation from both the American Academy of Neurology and the European Federation of Neurological Sciences in the treatment of dystonia. In many countries, it is the first-line treatment for CD. There are four types of toxin approved for the use in CD, three type A [OnabotulinumtoxinA (OnaBoNTA), AbobotulinumtoxinA (AboBoNTA), and Incobotulinumtoxin A (IncoBoNTA)] and one type B [RimabotulinumtoxinB (RimaBoNTB)]. Proper selection of affected muscles and dose of toxin are important parameters in successfully providing symptomatic treatment. Good response rate is defined as improvement of more than 25 % from baseline using the Toronto Western Torticollis Rating Scale. The most common side effect of chemodenervation with BoNT for CD is dysphagia.

Keywords: cervical dystonia, OnaBoNTA, AboBoNTA, IncoBoNTA, RimaBoNTB, botulinum toxin

1. Introduction

Cervical dystonia (CD) is a movement disorder characterized by involuntary contractions of cervical muscles causing abnormal head movements and postures, at times associated with head tremor and chronic pain [1, 2]. The prevalence of CD in the general population is estimated to vary from 0.006% from a clinic-based study in eight European countries to 0.4% in the USA, based on a consumer database survey [3, 4].

CD remains the most common of the focal dystonias [3, 5]. Classifications of CD include torticollis (turning or rotation of the head towards one side); laterocollis (tilting of the head towards one side); anterocollis (head and neck flexion); and retrocollis (head and neck extension) or a combination of these movements [1, 2]. The peak age of onset is around 41.8 years, although it can occur in all ages and is slightly more common in females [6]. Most cases of CD are idiopathic, and there is a family history in about 12% of cases [2]. It can also be secondary to trauma or musculoskeletal, spinal cord, intracranial, ocular, and vestibular disorders [7].

For objective rating of CD, the clinician has to use dedicated scales. Scoring at baseline, at the time of peak effect (approximately 1 month after injection) and before retreatment would allow the injectors to assess the outcome of the previous injection and make the necessary adjustment in the dosing and targeting in the next injection cycle [8]. The most frequently used instrument to assess the response to therapeutic interventions in patients with CD is the Toronto Western Spasmodic Torticollis Rating Scale (TWSTRS) [9]. The TWSTRS, together with the Cervical Dystonia Impact Scale (CDIP-58) and the Cervical Dystonia Questionnaire (CDQ-24), is "recommended" for CD, while the Functional Disability Questionnaire, the Tsui Scale and the Body Concept Scale have been rated as "suggested" [10].

2. Muscle selection

Upon diagnosis of CD, a proper clinical examination is warranted. One has to identify the primary muscles involved as opposed to compensatory activity as well as dose selection by the injector [8, 11].

The proper identification of muscles involved in CD cannot be overemphasized and requires an understanding of the different actions of the neck muscles. When examining the patient, dystonic muscles are best assessed when the neck is at rest or in submaximal contraction [8, 12]. More often than not, the dystonic muscles will show hypertrophy and are quite prominent. Superficial muscles are easily identified and palpated, making it easier to identify and inject. However, with deeper muscles, co-contraction of superficial muscles, or in certain cases where there is relative small muscle bulk, identification can be difficult.

Isolated postural deviations of the head occur in less than one-third of patients, while complex deviations occur in 66–80% of patients [1, 2]. There are generally four planes of movement in CD. However, most cases are compounded involving a combination of at least two movements, making muscle and dose selection more difficult.

Torticollis is when the neck turns from left to right or right to left along the horizontal axis in the coronal plane [22] (**Figure 1A**). Effector muscles for this action include the contralateral sternocleidomastoid and the ipsilateral splenius capitis, as well as other supporting neck muscles. In latercollis, the head tilts to one side along the vertical plane (**Figure 1B**). The movement is facilitated by the contractions of the ipsilateral splenius, sternocleidomastoid, scalene complex, levator scapulae, and posterior paravertebral muscles. In anterocollis, the head tilts forward (**Figure 1C**) and there is contraction of both sternocleidomastoids, scalene complex and the submental complex. Retrocollis is the opposite of the anterocollis, where the head tilts backwards (**Figure 1D**) and there are bilateral contractions of the splenius, deep paravertebral muscles, and upper trapezius. When compounded movements are present, muscle selection becomes more tedious and varying doses may prove beneficial. This includes identifying the more active dystonic muscles and preferentially giving these muscles a higher dose. In a patient who presents with both retrocollis and left torticollis (**Figure 1E**), the contralateral sternocleidomastoid and both splenius capitis muscles are chemodenervated, with the ipsilateral splenius receiving a higher dose than the contralateral counterpart. Another compound movement involves the lateral displacement of the neck along the horizontal axis (**Figure 1F**). A summary of involved muscles in the four general planes and some compound movements is seen in **Table 1**.

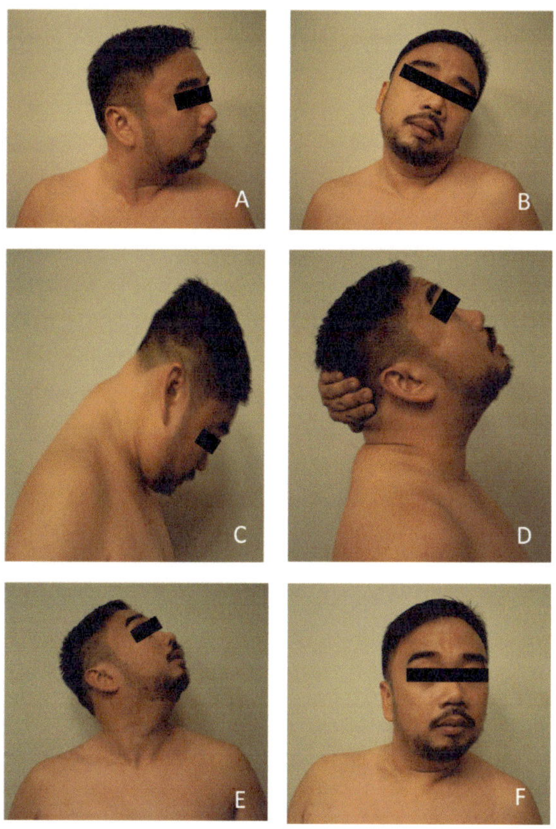

Figure 1. Different types of cervical dystonia. (A) Left torticollis, where the neck rotates to the left along the horizontal axis; (B) left laterocollis with the neck turned to the left along the vertical axis; (C) antecollis with the neck bent forward; (D) retrocollis with the neck bent backwards; (E) compound movement of both torticollis and retrocollis to the left with left shoulder elevation; and (F) lateral displacement of the neck along the horizontal axis.

	OnaBoNTA (Botox) [8, 41]	AboBoNTA (Dysport) [8, 42]	IncoBoNTA (Xeomin) [8, 43]	RimaBoNTB (NeuroBloc/Myobloc) [8, 44]
Torticollis				
CL SCM	20–50	40–120	20–50	1000–3000
CL Anterior scalene	5–30	20–100	5–30	500–2000
CL Middle scalene	5–30	20–100	5–30	500–2000
CL Semispinalis capitis	20–100	60–250	20–100	1000–2000
CL Levator scapulae	20–100	60–200	20–100	1000–2000
IP Splenius capitis	40–100	100–350	40–100	1000–4000
IP Longus capitis	15–30	20–60	15–30	ND
Laterocollis				
IP SCM	20–50	40–120	20–50	1000–3000
IP Anterior scalene	5–30	20–100	5–30	500–2000
IP Middle scalene	5–30	20–100	5–30	500–2000
IP Posterior scalene	5–30	20–100	5–30	500–2000
IP Splenius capitis	40–100	100–350	40–100	1000–4000
IP Semispinalis capitis	20–100	60–250	20–100	1000–2000
IP Levator scapulae	20–100	60–250	20–100	1000–2000
IP Trapezius	25–100	60–300	25–100	1000–4000
Retrocollis				
IP Splenius capitis	40–100	100–350	40–100	1000–4000
CL Splenius capitis	40–100	100–350	40–100	1000–4000
IP Semispinalis capitis	20–100	60–250	20–100	1000–2000
CL Semispinalis capitis	20–100	60–250	20–100	1000–2000
IP Trapezius	25–100	60–300	25–100	1000–4000
CL Trapezius	25–100	60–300	25–100	1000–4000
Anterocollis				
IP SCM	20–50	40–120	20–50	1000–3000
CL SCM	20–50	40–120	20–50	1000–3000
IP Longus collis	15–30	20–60	15–30	ND
CL Longus collis	15–30	20–60	15–30	ND
IP Anterior scalene	5–30	20–100	5–30	500–2000
CL Anterior scalene	5–30	20–100	5–30	500–2000

IP: ipsilateral; CL: contralateral; ND: No Data; SCM: sternocleidomastoid.

Table 1. Target muscles and dose of BoNT for CD.

The use of equipment such as electromyography (EMG), ultrasonography, endoscopic/fluoroscopic, and even computed tomography guidance may help to locate the target muscles and thus lessen occurrence of unintended weakness of uninjected muscles [8, 13–16]. This is discussed in another chapter.

3. Treatment of cervical dystonia

The treatment of CD was initially limited to oral medication and eventually surgery.

These medications include anticholinergics, benzodiazepines, and antispasticity medications [17]. As much as 40% of patients reported improvement with trihexyphenidyl [18, 19]. However, these medications are often of limited benefit due to systemic side effects. Surgery with deep brain stimulation or selective peripheral denervation surgery for CD has shown inconsistent results [20–23].

The efficacy of Botulinum toxin (BoNT) has been demonstrated, warranting both European Federation of Neurological Societies (EFNS) and the American Association of Neurology (AAN) level A recommendations as first-line treatment [24, 25]. BoNT has been approved for use in many countries and remains the treatment of choice for CD [8, 18, 26, 27]. Recent studies also provided level A evidence supporting for the treatment of CD [28].

In its updated guideline, the AAN has now differentiated the different serotypes/preparations of BoNT and its level of evidence for CD: AboBoNTA and RimaBoNTB should be offered (Level A) while OnaBoNTA and IncoBoNTA should be considered (Level B), as options for the treatment of CD [26].

Reviews of BoNT treatment for CD suggest that 70–90% of patients derive symptomatic benefit from BoNT with at least one injection [29–31]. In a meta-analysis (8 trials with 361 patients using OnaBoNTA; 5 trials with 319 patients using AboBoNTA), it was shown that there was a statistically and clinically significant improvement on objective rating scales and subjective rating scales as well as for pain relief in subjective scales [7]. The same was also seen in a real-world design study (1046 patients) showing robust improvement in clinical ratings as measured via both physician- and subject-reported outcomes and excellent tolerability following OnaBoNTA treatment of CD [30].

There is no consensus on the duration of effect of the various BoNT in the treatment of CD. The minimum treatment duration was 7.8 ± 1.4 weeks, and maximum treatment duration was 21.0 ± 3.9 weeks [32]. Only 49.3% of patients rated the duration of response of >12 weeks for all BoNTA preparations [33]. In a comparative study of BoNT preparations for the treatment of CD, a significant difference in overall duration of effect was seen between the various groups with a mean duration of 104.3 days for the current formulation of OnaBoNTA, 75.7 days for AboBoNTA, and 91.2 days for RimaBoNTB [34].

OnaBoNTA and IncoBoNTA have comparable efficacies with a 1:1 conversion ratio and have demonstrated therapeutic equivalence in different indications including CD. An OnaBoNTA to AboBoNTA conversion ratio of 1:3, or even less, should be considered the most appropriate [35–38]. It is interesting that an Asian study found a clinical equivalent ratio of 1:2.5 [39]. A robust conversion factor of estimating the equivalent doses of BoNTA and Botulinum toxin B (BoNTB) remains to be tested in the clinics.

The injection interval of BoNT for the treatment of CD is typically 3–4 months in most clinical practices [40]. In one study (59 subjects), the inter-injection interval was 15.4 ± 3.4 weeks [32].

In the CD-PROBE registry, the mean time between treatments increased from 14.6 ± 4.1 weeks following treatment session 1 to 15.1 ± 5.2 weeks after treatment session 2 [30].

A single injection cycle of BoNT is effective and safe for treating CD, and further injection cycles continue to work for most patients [7].

4. Botulinum toxin therapy dosing

The appropriate dose given to the target muscles is equally important in a successful injection session. There are several types of BoNTs available; however, only four types have been approved for use in CD: three type A and one type B toxin. The approved toxins for use are OnaBoNTA (Botox), AboBoNTA (Dysport), IncoBoNTA (Xeomin), and RimaBoNTB (Neuro-Bloc/Myobloc). Although three of these are type A toxins, they are not equivalent. A summary of the common muscles to be injected according to the type of CD and its BoNT doses is presented in **Table 1**. Generally, in the initial treatment session, each muscle injected should not exceed 200 units for OnaBoNTA and IncoBoNTA, 500 units for AboBoNTA, and 5000 units for RimaBoNTB. The total dose given per patient per session should also not exceed 400 units for OnaBoNTA and IncoBoNTA, 1000 units for AboBoNTA, and 10,000 units for RimaBoNTB [8, 36].

5. Challenges with BoNT therapy

Responders to BoNT therapy is based on four criteria: magnitude of effect defined as more than 25% improvement in the TWSTRS, at least 12-week duration of effect as reported by the patient, tolerability defined as absence of severe related adverse events, and subjective perception of improvement [33].

For nonresponders, the clinician has to know whether the patient is a primary or secondary nonresponder or is a poor responder (treatment failure) [45]. Common determinants for an unsuccessful chemodenervation session/poor responder include suboptimal doses, suboptimal muscle targeting, intolerable side effects, and complex movement patterns, discordant expectations, and an incorrect diagnosis [46].

Although BoNTA resistance is a recognized entity, secondary nonresponse maybe due to other factors including the underlying severity of the CD [27, 47]. When confronted with these situations, it is prudent to investigate with neuroimaging techniques before the next injection session. A CT scan of the neck to visualize the cervical spine may help define the nature of dystonia. Employing this imaging technique is based on the new phenomenological classification for CD by Reichel with reference to the position of the cervical vertebrae from the head position. Torticollis and laterocollis involves the same angle of rotation from across all cervical vertebrae; however, when there is torticaput or laterocaput, the base of the skull and C1 are on the same degree of rotation but differ from the rest of the cervical spine [48, 49]. The challenge for the injector confronted with these movements is to target deeper and smaller muscles. In patients with torticaput, it has been shown that 73% of cases involve the obliquus capitis inferior [49]. It is important to keep this in mind and to discuss the planned session with the patient including expected results to optimize treatment [8].

6. Adverse events

BoNT has a favorable safety profile. There is often a delicate balance to be found between achieving optimal efficacy and avoiding adverse events (AEs) [50]. The AEs of BoNT treatment are usually mild and self-limiting and similar in both nature and severity between the different formulations [8]. However, in some cases the outcome is disappointing or side effects occur. This can be due to the fact that either the target muscles were not injected accurately or unintended weakness of nontarget muscles occurred [15].

The most common AEs related to BoNT type A are as follows: dysphagia; neck muscle weakness; injection site pain; and "flu-like" symptoms [51]. AEs of BoNT type A are dose-related and mostly due to contiguous or distant spread of toxin. Therefore, it is important that injections are located precisely so that potential spread of toxin is minimized.

A meta-analysis of 36 randomized controlled studies reported AEs in 25% (353/1425) of the OnaBoNTA-treated patient versus 15% (133/884) in controls [52].

In a systematic review of the various preparations of BoNT in the treatment of CD, a significantly higher rate of dysphagia and positive dose-related effect were reported with AboBoNTA compared with the current formulation of OnaBoNTA or RimaBoNTB [34]. However, in another study, it was mentioned that the dysphagia did not appear to be dose- or treatment cycle-related [53].

In the CD-PROBE registry, 185 patients (17.8%) given OnaBoNTA experienced treatment-related adverse events. The most common events were weakness (6.9%, 185 subjects), dysphagia (6.2%, 65 subjects), and neck pain (2.3%, 24 subjects) [30].

For IncoBoNTA, the most frequently reported adverse events were dysphagia, neck pain, and muscle weakness which were usually mild [54].

Dry mouth was reported more frequently in the studies of RimaBoNTB compared to the formulations of BoNT type A; however, a dose-related effect was not seen with RimaBoNTB [34].

Most of these complications resolve spontaneously, usually within 2 weeks. Dysphagia was most frequently related to bilateral injection into sternocleidomastoid muscles [55, 56]. Measures to minimize these adverse events include always using the lowest effective dose.

7. Conclusion

BoNT remains the treatment of choice for CD. There are three BoNT type A and one BoNT type B formulations that are currently approved, and each has its own unique pharmacologic properties that may confer different side effect profiles, duration of therapeutic effects, and dosing recommendations [57,58].

A number of factors need to be considered in BoNT treatment. These include the correct diagnosis of CD, number and selection of neck and adjacent muscles to inject, the amount dose to use, and the length of intervals of reinjection. One has to remember that each patient will have to be individually assessed for dose and response optimization.

Acknowledgements

The authors wish to thank Dr. Jennifer Justice Manzano for her help.

Author details

Roland Dominic G. Jamora[1,2*] and Anthony N. Piano[3]

*Address all correspondence to: rgjamora@up.edu.ph

1 Department of Neurosciences, College of Medicine – Philippine General Hospital, University of the Philippines Manila, Manila, Philippines

2 Movement Disorders Service and Section of Adult Neurology, Institute for Neurosciences, St. Luke's Medical Center, Quezon City and Global City, Philippines

3 Movement Disorders Clinic and Section of Neurology, Department of Medicine, The Medical City, Pasig City, Philippines

References

[1] Chan J, Brin MF, Fahn S. Idiopathic cervical dystonia: clinical characteristics. Mov Disord. 1991;6:119–126. doi:http://dx.doi.org/10.1002/mds.870060206

[2] Jankovic J, Leder S, Warner D, Schwartz K. Cervical dystonia: clinical findings and associated movement disorders. Neurology. 1991;41:1088–1091. doi:http://dx.doi.org/10.1212/WNL.41.7.1088

[3] Epidemiological Study of Dystonia in Europe (ESDE) Collaborative Group. A prevalence study of primary dystonia in eight European countries. J Neurol. 2000;247:787–792. doi:http://dx.doi.org/10.1007/s004150070094

[4] Jankovic J, Tsui J, Bergeron C. Prevalence of cervical dystonia and spasmodic torticollis in the United States general population. Parkinsonism Relat Disord. 2007;13:411–416. doi:http://dx.doi.org/10.1016/j.parkreldis.2007.02. 005

[5] Jamora RD, Tan AK, Tan LC. A 9-year review of dystonia from a movement disorders clinic in Singapore. Eur J Neurol. 2006;13:77–81. doi:10.1111/j.1468-1331.2006.01150.x

[6] Kessler KR, Skutta M, Benecke R. Long-term treatment of cervical dystonia with botulinum toxin A: efficacy, safety, and antibody frequency. German Dystonia Study Group. J Neurol. 1999;246:265–274. doi:10.1007/s004150050345

[7] Costa J, Espírito-Santo C, Borges A, Ferreira J, Coelho M, Moore P, Sampaio C. Botulinum toxin type A therapy for cervical dystonia. Cochrane Database Syst Rev. 2005;(1): CD003633. doi:10.1002/14651858.CD003633.pub2

[8] Albanese A, Abbruzzese G, Dressler D, Duzynski W, Khatkova S, Marti MJ, Mir P, Montecucco C, Moro E, Pinter M, Relja M, Roze E, Skogseid IM, Timerbaeva S, Tzoulis C. Practical guidance for CD management involving treatment of botulinum toxin: a consensus statement. J Neurol. 2015;262:2201–2213. doi:10.1007/s00415-015-7703-x

[9] Comella CL, Stebbins GT, Goetz CG, Chmura TA, Bressman SB, Lang AE. Teaching tape for the motor section of the Toronto Western Spasmodic Torticollis Scale. Mov Disord. 1997;12:570–575. doi:10.1002/mds.870120414

[10] Albanese A, Sorbo FD, Comella C, Jinnah HA, Mink JW, Post B, Vidailhet M, Volkmann J, Warner TT, Leentjens AF, Martinez-Martin P, Stebbins GT, Goetz CG, Schrag A. Dystonia rating scale: critique and recommendations. Mov Disord. 2013;28:874–883. doi:10.1002/mds.25579

[11] Jankovic J. Treatment of cervical dystonia with botulinum toxin. Mov Disord. 2004;19:S109-S115. DOI:10.1002/mds.20024

[12] De Bruijn E, Nijmeijer SW, Forbes PA, Koelman JH, van der Helm FC, Tijssen MA, Happee R. Improved identification of dystonic cervical muscles via abnormal muscle activity during isometric contractions. J Neurol Sci. 2015;354:10–16. doi:10.1016/j.jns.2015.03.047

[13] Allison SK, Odderson IR. Ultrasound and electromyography guidance for injection of the longus colli with botulinum toxin for the treatment of cervical dystonia. Ultrasound Q. 2016; doi:10.1097/RUQ.0000000000000226

[14] Grigoriu Al, Dinomais M, Remy-Neris O, Brochard S. Impact of injection-guiding techniques on the effectiveness of botulinum toxin for the treatment of focal spasticity and dystonia: a systematic review. Arch Phys Med Rehabil. 2015;96:2067–2078. doi: 10.1016/j.apmr.2015.05.002

[15] Schramm A, Baumer T, Fietzek U, Heitmann S, Walter U, Jost WH. Relevance of sonography for botulinum toxin treatment of cervical dystonia: an expert statement. J Neural Transm (Vienna). 2015;122:1457–1463. doi:10.1007/s00702-014-1356-2

[16] Lim EC, Quek AM, Seet RC. Accurate targeting of botulinum toxin injections: how to and why. Parkinsonism Relat Disord. 2011;17:S34-S39. doi:10.1016/j.parkreldis. 2011.06.016

[17] Bressman SB. Dystonia update. Clin Neuropharmacol. 2000;23:239–251

[18] Brans JW, Lindeboom R, Snoek JW, Zwarts MJ, van Weerden TW, Brunt ER, van Hilten JJ, van der Kamp W, Prins MH, Speelman JD. Botulinum toxin versus trihexyphenidyl in cervical dystonia: a prospective, randomized, double-blind controlled trial. Neurology.1996;46:1066–1072. doi:10.1212/WNL.46.4.1066

[19] Balash Y, Giladi N. Efficacy of pharmacological treatment of dystonia: evidence-based review including meta-analysis of the effect of botulinum toxin and other cure options. Eur J Neurol. 2004;11:361–370. doi:10.1111/j.1468-1331.2004.00845.x

[20] Tagliati M, Krack P, Volkmann J, Aziz T, Krauss JK, Kupsch A, Vidailhet AM. Long-term management of DBS in dystonia: response to stimulation, adverse events, battery changes, and special considerations. Mov Disord. 2011;26:S54-S62. doi:10.1002/mds. 23535

[21] Ford B, Louis ED, Greene P, Fahn S. Outcome of selective ramisectomy for botulinum toxin resistant torticollis. J Neurol Neurosurg Psychiatry. 1998;65:472–478. doi:10.1136/ jnnp.65.4.472

[22] Münchau A, Palmer JD, Dressler D, O'Sullivan JD, Tsang KL, Jahanshahi M, Quinn NP, Lees AJ, Bhatia KP. Prospective study of selective peripheral denervation for botulinum-toxin resistant patients with cervical dystonia. Brain. 2001;124:769–783. doi:http:// dx.doi.org/10.1093/brain/124.4.769

[23] Braun V, Richter HP. Selective peripheral denervation for spasmodic torticollis: 13-year experience with 155 patients. J Neurosurg. 2002;97:207–212.

[24] Simpson DM, Blitzer A, Brashear A, Comella C, Dubinsky R, Hallett M, Jankovic J, Karp B, Ludlow CL, Miyasaki JM, Naumann M, So Y. Assessment: botulinum neurotoxin for the treatment of movement disorders (an evidence-based review): report of the Therapeutics and Technology Assessment Subcommittee of the American Academy of Neurology. Neurology. 2008;70:1699–1706. doi:http://dx. doi.org/10.1212/01.wnl. 0000311389.26145.95

[25] Albanese A, Barnes MP, Bhatia KP, Fernandez-Alvarez E, Filippini G, Gasser T, Krauss JK, Newton A, Rektor I, Savoiardo M, Valls-Solè J. A systematic review on the diagnosis and treatment of primary (idiopathic) dystonia and dystonia plus syndromes: report of an EFNS/MDS-ES task force. Eur J Neurol. 2006;13:433–444. doi:10.1111/j.1468-1331.2006.01537.x

[26] Simpson DM, Hallett M, Ashman EJ, Comella CL, Green MW, Gronseth GS, Armstrong MJ, Gloss D, Potrebic S, Jankovic J, Karp BP, Naumann M, So YT, Yablon SA. Practice guideline update summary: botulinum neurotoxin for the treatment of blepharospasm, cervical dystonia, adult spasticity, and headache. Report of the Guideline Development Subcommittee of the American Academy of Neurology. Neurology. 2016;86:1–9. doi:http:// dx. doi. org/ 10. 1212/ WNL. 0000000000002560

[27] Bledsoe IO, Comella CL. Botulinum toxin treatment of cervical dystonia. Semin Neurol. 2016;36:47–53. doi:http://dx.doi.org/ 10.1055/s-0035-1571210

[28] Hallett M, Albanese A, Dressler D, Segal KR, Simpson DM, Truong D, Jankovic J. Evidence-based review and assessment of botulinum neurotoxin for the treatment of movement disorders. Toxicon. 2013;67:94–114

[29] Swope D, Barbano R. Treatment recommendations and practical applications of botulinum toxin treatment of cervical dystonia. Neurol Clin. 2008;26:54–65. doi:http://dx.doi.org/10.1016/S0733-8619(08)80005-9

[30] Jankovic J, Adler CH, Charles D, Comella C, Stacy M, Schwarts M, Adams AM, Brin MF. Primary results from the Cervical Dystonia Patient Registry for Observation of Onabotulinumtoxin A Efficacy (CD PROBE). J Neurol Sci. 2015;349:84–93. doi:10.1016/j.jns.2014.12.030

[31] Zoons E, Dijkgraaf MG, Dijk JM, van Schaik IN, Tijssen MA. Botulinum toxin as treatment for focal dystonia: a systematic review of the pharmaco-therapeutic and pharmaco-economic value. J Neurol. 2012;259:2519–2526. doi:http://dx.doi.org/10.1007/s00415-012-6510-x

[32] Dressler D, Tacik P, Saberi FA. Botulinum toxin therapy of cervical dystonia. J Neural Transm (Vienna). 2015;122:297–300. doi:10.1007/s00702-014-1253-8

[33] Misra VP, Ehler E, Zakine B, Maisonobe P, Simonetta-Moreau M; INTEREST IN CD group. Factors influencing response to Botulinum toxin type A in patients with idiopathic cervical dystonia: results from an international observational study. BMJ Open. 2012;2(3).pii: e000881. doi:10.1136/bmjopen-2012-000881

[34] Chapman MA, Barron R, Tanis DC, Gill CE, Charles PD. Comparison of botulinum neurotoxin preparations for the treatment of cervical dystonia. Clin Ther. 2007;29:1325–1337. doi:http://dx.doi.org/10.1016/j.clinthera.2007.07.020

[35] Scaglione F. Conversion ratio between Botox, Dysport, and Xeomin in clinical practice. Toxins (Basel). 2016;8(3). pii: E65. doi:10.3390/toxins8030065

[36] Poewe W, Deuschl G, Nebe A, Feifel E, Wissel J, Benecke R, Kressler KR, Ceballos? Baumann AO, Ohly A, Oertel W, Ku?niget G. What is the optimal dose of botulinum toxin A in the treatment of cervical dystonia? Results of a double blind, placebo controlled, dose ranging study using Dysport. J Neurol Neurosurg Psychiatry. 1998;64:13-17. doi:10.1136/jnnp.64.1.13

[37] Odergren T, Hjalatason H, Kaakkola S, Solders G, Hanko J, Fehling C, Marttila RJ, Lundh H, Gedin S, Westergren I, Richardson A, Dott C, Cohen H. A double blind, randomised, parallel group study to investigate the dose equivalence of Dysport and Botox in the treatment of cervical dystonia. J Neurol Neurosurg Psychiatry. 1998;64:6-12. doi:10.1136/jnnp.64.1.6

[38] Ranoux D, Gury C, Fondarai J, Mas JL, Zuberet M. Respective potencies of Botox and Dysport: a double?blind, randomized, cross?over study in cervical dystonia. J Neurol Neurosurg Psychiatry. 2002;72:459-462. doi:10.1136/jnnp.72.4.459

[39] Yun JY, Kim JW, Kim HT, Chung SJ, Kim JM, Cho JW, Lee JY, Lee HN, You S, Oh E, Jeong H, Kim YE, Kim HJ, Lee WY, Jeon BS. Dysport and Botox at a ratio of 2.5:1 units in cervical dystonia: a double?blind, randomized study. Mov Disord. 2015;30:206-213. doi:10.1002/mds. 26085

[40] Marsh WA, Monroe DM, Brin MF, Gallagher CJ. Systematic review and meta-analysis of the duration of clinical effect of onabotulinumtoxinA in cervical dystonia. BMC Neurol. 2014;14:91. doi:10.1186/1471-2377-14-91

[41] Botox 100 Units. Available from: http:www.medicine.org.uk/emc/medicine/112 [Accessed: 2016-05-14]

[42] Dysport 300 Units. Available from: http:www.medicine.org.uk/emc/medicine/870. [Accessed: 2016-05-14]

[43] Xeomin 100 Units powder for solution for injection. Available from: http:www.medicine.org.uk/emc/medicine/20666 [Accessed: 2016-05-14]

[44] NeuroBloc 5000 U/ml solution for injection. Available from: http:www.medicine.org.uk/emc/medicine/20568/SPC [Accessed: 2016-05-14]

[45] Marion MH, Humberstone M, Grunewald R, Wimalaratna S. British Neurotoxin Network recommendations for managing cervical dystonia in patients with a poor response to botulinum toxin. Pract Neurol. 2016;16:288-295. doi: 10.1136/practneurol-2015-001335

[46] Jinnah HA, Goodmann E, Rosen AR, Evatt M, Freeman A, Factor S. Botulinum toxin treatment failures in cervical dystonia: causes, management, and outcomes. J Neurol. 2016;263:1188-1194. doi:10.1007/s00415-016-8136-x

[47] Ferreira JJ, Colosimo C, Bhidayasiri R, Marti MJ, Maisonobe P, Om S. Factors influencing secondary non-response to botulinum toxin type A injections in cervical dystonia. Parkinsonism Relat Disord. 2015;21:111–115. doi:10.1016/j.parkreldis.2014.09.034

[48] Reichel G. Dystonias of the Neck: clinico-radiologic correlations. In: RL Rosales (Editor). Dystonia: The Many Facets. (Intech Open Access Publishers, Croatia), 2012, ISBN: 978-953-307-1116-8 (www.intechopen.com) (pp 17–32)

[49] Reichel G. Cervical dystonia: a new phenomenological classification for botulinum toxin therapy. Basal Ganglia. 20111:5-12. doi: 10.1016/j.baga.2011.01.001

[50] Brashear A. Botulinum toxin type A in the treatment of patients with cervical dystonia. Biologics. 2009;3:1–7. doi:http://dx.doi.org/10.2147/BTT.S3113

[51] Truong D. Botulinum toxins in the treatment of primary focal dystonias. J Neurol Sci. 2012;316:9–14. doi:10.1016/j.jns.2012.01.019

[52] Naumann M, Jankovic J. Safety of botulinum toxin type A: a systematic review and meta-analysis. Curr Med Res Opin. 2004;20:981–990. doi:10.1185/030079904125003962

[53] Truong D, Brodsky M, Lew M, Brashear A, Jankovic J, Molho E, Orlova O, Timerbaeva S; Global Dysport Cervical Dystonia Study Group. Long-term efficacy and safety of botulinum toxin type A (Dysport) in cervical dystonia. Parkinsonism Relat Disord. 2010;16(5): 316–323. doi:10.1016/j.parkreldis.2010.03.002

[54] Comella CL, Jankovic J, Truong DD, Hanschmann A, Grafe S; U.S. XEOMIN Cervical Dystonia Study Group. Efficacy and safety of IncobotulinumtoxinA (NT 201, XEOMIN®, botulinum neurotoxin type A, without accessory proteins) in patients with cervical dystonia. J Neurol Sci. 2011;308:103–109. doi:10.1016/j.jns.2011.05.041

[55] Jankovic J. Schwartz KS. Clinical correlates of response to botulinum toxin injections. Arch Neurol. 1991;48:1253–1256. doi:10.1001/archneur.1991.00530240057020

[56] Comella Cl, Tanner CM, DeFoor-Hill L, Smith C. Dysphagia after botulinum toxin injections for spasmodic torticollis. Clinical and radiologic findings. Neurology. 1992;42:1307–1310. doi:10.1212/WNL.42.7.1307

[57] Mills RR, Pagan FL. Patient considerations in the treatment of cervical dystonia: focus on botulinum toxin A. Patient Prefer Adherence. 2015;9:725–731. doi:10.2147/PPA.S75459

[58] Han Y, Stevens AL, Dashtipour K, Hauser RA, Mari Z. A mixed treatment comparison to compare the efficacy and safety of botulinum toxin treatments for cervical dystonia. J Neurol. 2016;263:772–780. doi 10.1007/s00415-016-8050-2

Chapter 7

What Clinical Strategies are Applied for Botulinum Toxin Injection in the Oromandibular Region?

Merete Bakke, Torben Dalager and Eigild Møller

Additional information is available at the end of the chapter

http://dx.doi.org/10.5772/64271

Abstract

Botulinum neurotoxin (BoNT) inhibits the release of acetylcholine from cholinergic nerve terminals in muscles or salivary glands. With reduced activation, the muscle activity or secretion decreases. Indications for medical, non-cosmetic use of BoNT in the orofacial area include among others oromandibular dystonia, painful masseter hypertrophy, Frey's syndrome, and severe drooling. The chapter covers anamnestic characteristics of these conditions as well as clinical, electromyographic (EMG) and laboratory findings, treatment methods with guided injections, and outcome from systematic treatment controls and follow-up examinations.

Keywords: dystonia, drooling, Frey's syndrome, masticatory muscles, salivary glands

1. Introduction

There are a limited number of publications concerning botulinum neurotoxin (BoNT) treatment in the oromandibular region, probably due to an overlap between the working areas for dentists and medical specialists. This chapter presents various neurological and neuromuscular conditions that may benefit from treatment with BoNT, and strategies developed for such treatment based on the collaboration between dental, neurological, and neurophysiological specialists in hospitals and university clinics.

In addition to its action at cholinergic motor endings, acetylcholine is also an important neurotransmitter in the autonomic nervous system. Thus, BoNT can be injected into muscles and salivary glands to achieve therapeutic benefit in a large range of clinical conditions in the oromandibular region such as dystonia, spasticity, and drooling. With reduced or blocked release of acetylcholine, the signals from the nervous system to the muscles or glands are decreased. This results in a temporary functional denervation of the muscle fibers with inhibition of the contractions and paralysis, and a temporary functional denervation of the salivary glands with reduced secretion. In the oromandibular region with small muscle groups, vital functions, and delicate anatomical structures, precise injection of the BoNT is crucial. Diffusion at injection site and spread to unintended areas may lead to significant although temporary discomfort. Such problems are most often swallowing difficulties due to effect on adjacent muscle groups or dry mouth from displacement into salivary glands. Therefore, it is strongly advocated to use guidance of the injections by EMG and/or ultrasonography to avoid off-target side effects and to secure effective placing of BoNT.

The latency for the full effect on the muscles after injection of BoNT is about a week, and the effect is optimal within the first 1.5–2 months. Since neuromuscular transmission regenerates slowly, muscle function is restored and the effect ceased after 3–6 months. Therefore, BoNT treatments are typically repeated up to three to four times per year. Inhibition of the release of acetylcholine from the postganglionic parasympathetic nerve ending to the salivary glands and the effect on the salivary secretions has a similar course [1, 2, 21]. BoNT/A, onabotulinumtoxinA (A/Ona), abobotulinumtoxinA (A/Abo), incobotulinumtoxinA (A/Inco), and BoNT/B, rimabotulinumtoxinB (B/Rima) are used for the treatment of muscles and salivary glands. There may be a small risk of developing antibodies and immunity by repeated treatments with the same type of BoNT. Therefore, it is generally recommended to have an interval of at least 3 months between treatments. If the patient seems to develop resistance to one type of BoNT, so that treatment is ineffective, the other is attempted [1].

Unlike other drugs, there is no direct correlation between the dosage units for the various compositions of BoNT. Depending on the preparation, there may be up to 50-fold difference in the number of units for the same treatment. Thus, the recommended dose is specific to the individual preparations. Storage and dilution differ also for the different compositions. Therefore, instructions for each preparation must be reviewed carefully to avoid mistakes, and the substance for injection must be diluted with saline corresponding to the needed units and the target for the treatment.

2. Oromandibular muscles

BoNT/A is the preferred choice for the muscles in the oromandibular region [3]. In most cases, the indication for such treatment is based on electromyographic (EMG) examination with bipolar surface electrodes and/or concentric needle electrodes. The indication for treating a muscle is abnormally increased spontaneous activity. This is defined partly as a mean level significantly above the reference for postural activity and partly as an activity pattern with more than 100 turns per second [4]. The dose depends on the activity and volume of the muscles (**Figure 1**) [1, 5–7]. When treating a muscle in a patient for the first time, the dose is usually low. In the following treatments, it is adjusted individually corresponding to the effect. This strategy not only reduces the possibility of side effects but also minimizes the cost.

http://dx.doi.org/10.5772/64271

Oromandibular muscles	Maximal voluntary contraction	Units of A/Ona or A/Inco
Temporalis		
Masseter	Jaw closing	10-45
Medial pterygoid		
Anterior digastric	Jaw opening	5-10
Lateral pterygoid	Jaw opening, side movement and protrusion	10-45
Orbicularis oris	Lip pursing	5-10

Figure 1. Oromandibular muscles, their maximal activation, and recommended doses of BoNT/A. Units are shown for one muscle in one side and for the orbicularis oris muscle for each side of the upper and lower part of the lip. It is advisable to start treatment with a low dose when treating a muscle in a patient for the first time. The patient should be informed that injections into the digastric muscle may give temporary swallowing difficulties. A/Ona: onabotulinumtoxinA and A/Inco: incobotulinumtoxinA. For A/Abo (abobotulinumtoxinA) is the dose probably 2.5 times higher [7].

The BoNT is injected as a bolus with cannulated electrodes and EMG guidance. One injection site is normally sufficient in the oromandibular muscles. If unfamiliar with the possible injection site in the oromandibular muscles, the procedures become easier after checking the locations and anatomic details of the targeted muscles, and if possible, to palpate them during maximal voluntary contraction (see **Figure 1**).

The site for the percutaneous injection into the masseter is the lower half of the superficial part, for the anterior voluminous part of the temporalis muscle, for the medial pterygoid muscle on the medial side of the ramus above its fusion with the masseter to form a common tendinous sling, and for the anterior belly of the digastric muscle. With respect to the orbicularis oris muscles, the injections are placed in the protruding parts but just above (upper lip) or below (lower lip) the carmine margin of the lip. The lateral (external) pterygoid is best approached intraorally to have direct access for palpation and injection. The direction of the needle insertion is posteriorly and slightly laterally in parallel with the buccal surfaces of the maxillary molars. Sometimes a more problematic percutaneous approach for the lateral pterygoid muscle is used with injection in front of the tragus and the mandibular condyle. However, with the intraoral approach, there is less vasculature encountered, and the risk of injecting several branches of the trigeminal and facial nerves is reduced, as well as injecting the parotid gland (that may lead to mouth dryness) [8]. In addition, the intraoral approach allows recording during chewing as well as opening and lateral movements of the mandible [9]; (**Figure 1**). When the cannulated electrode is inserted, the position is verified by the presence of well-defined sharp spikes with high EMG amplitude during posture. Subsequently, the level of maximal activity is recorded to ascertain a normal interference pattern during maximal effort of the muscle, that is, strong biting, jaw opening, lateral jaw movement, or pursing of the lips.

2.1. Temporomandibular disorders (TMD)

As TMDs are the most common disorders in the oromandibular region, they should be mentioned shortly. The prevalence in the adult population is 8–15% [10]. TMD are recognized as a group of musculoskeletal and neuromuscular conditions that involve the temporomandibular joints, the masticatory muscles, and associated tissues [11]. The signs and symptoms of TMD are orofacial pain and impaired jaw function, and they may be confused with other conditions in the orofacial region. However, in contrast to the other conditions mentioned in this chapter, BoNT treatment does not seem to have a significant role in the treatment of TMD and episodic tension headaches, and evidence on the effect of BoNT on most orofacial pain conditions is lacking [12, 13].

2.2. Painful bilateral masseter hypertrophy

Benign masseter hypertrophy is characterized by a soft swelling near the angle of the mandible. It is relatively uncommon and may occur unilaterally or bilaterally [14].The swelling can be so prominent that it is considered cosmetically disfiguring. Occasionally, there are also pain symptoms. The condition may be associated with clenching and bruxism but often it is idiopathic. Diagnosis of masseter hypertrophy should not be based on the clinical findings alone as differential diagnoses are conditions such as tumors in the muscle and parotid gland. The diagnosis should be supported by imaging with ultrasonic or magnetic resonance scanning. Various treatment options have been reported including surgical reduction, while injection of BoNT/A into the masseter muscle represents a less invasive modality [15, 16].

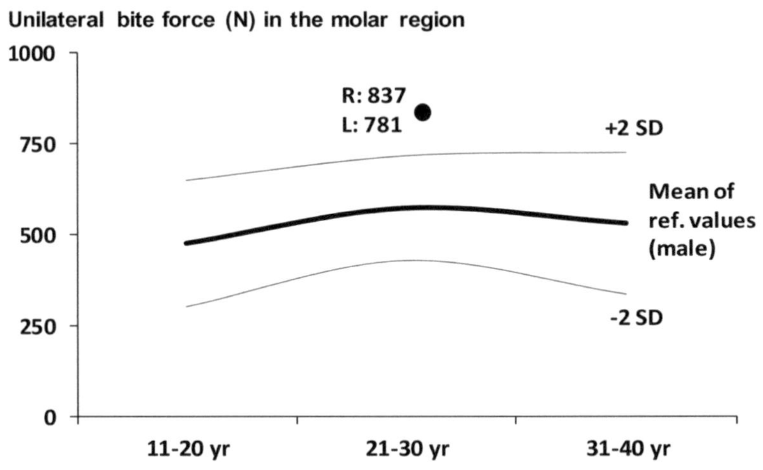

Figure 2. Increased bite force in a young man with painful masseter hypertrophy. Recording of maximum unilateral clenching force during 1–2 s biting on a strain-gauge transducer in the right and left molar region before treatment with indications of reference values (M and SD; average of stored peak values) [17].

To illustrate the treatment strategy with BoNT for this condition, a case with a 24-year-old male student is presented. He developed increasing masseter hypertrophy through some years with high mental stress. The condition was painful and associated with a feeling of jaw tension. In

http://dx.doi.org/10.5772/64271

addition, he reported sleep bruxism. The hypertrophy was documented by ultrasonic scanning of the muscle structure. Examinations of the muscle function with bite-force measurements and EMG of the masseter muscles showed increased values (**Figure 2**). The increased muscle volume was ascribed to his sleep bruxism, based on reports from his companions, and as the dental attrition was greater than might be expected from his age. Treatment was performed with BoNT/A injections into the masseter muscles. At the first treatment, the dose was low, 20 units A/Ona in each masseter. The intramuscular injections were repeated twice with 3–4 months intervals with 30 units A/Ona in each masseter to a total of three treatment series. No further BoNT treatment was necessary as the pain and the thickness of the muscles were reduced (**Figure 3A** and **B**). After the BoNT treatments, a bite splint was provided to reduce further dental attrition as he still had episodes with grinding of his teeth during sleep.

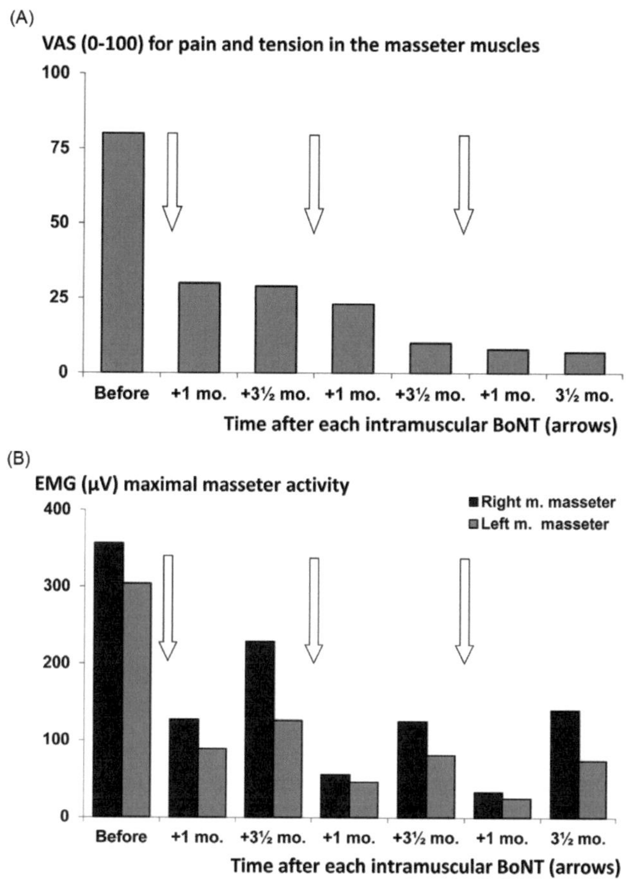

Figure 3. Jaw pain and muscle activity in a young man with painful masseter hypertrophy treated with intramuscular BoNT injection. (A) Jaw pain and feelings of jaw tension recorded on horizontal visual analog scales (VAS) before treatment and at controls during the treatment period. (B) Recordings with surface electromyography from right and left masseter muscles during maximum biting in the intercuspal position measured before treatment and at controls during the treatment period. Reference value is M: 250 μV, SD: 180 μV (bipolar electrodes, mean voltage; custom-designed 8-channel EMG system; Electromyographic Laboratory, Dept. of Odontology, University of Copenhagen) [18].

2.3. Oromandibular dystonia (OMD)

OMD is a rare focal neurological disorder affecting the lower part of the face and jaws. It is characterized by sustained or repetitive involuntary jaw and tongue movements and facial grimacing, caused by involuntary activity of the masticatory, facial, pharyngeal, lingual, and lip muscles [19]. The dystonic activity may look similar to idiopathic sleep bruxism but it usually ceases during sleep. Dystonia is thought to be derived from dysfunction of the basal ganglia, and the excess movements to be due to loss of inhibitory motor control. Neurophysiologic and neuroimaging studies have shown abnormalities at cortical and subcortical levels, probably reflecting a dysfunction in the basal ganglia-thalamo-cortical circuits. However, peripheral mechanisms and abnormal sensorimotor integration or somatosensory dysfunction may occur in dystonia and aggravate the disorder [20].

OMD is typically classified as jaw opening, jaw closing, jaw deviating, or lingual dystonia (tongue protrusion or curling) or combinations of these [8]. The combination of OMD, blepharospasms (sustained, forced, involuntary closing of the eyelids), and dystonic movements of the upper face is known as Meige's syndrome [6]. OMD often interferes with normal orofacial function, such as chewing and control of food bolus, swallowing, and verbal and nonverbal communication. EMG recordings have shown high spontaneous and deviating masticatory muscle activity with co-contractions of antagonists and loss of rhythmicity during chewing [5, 19]. Depending on the subtype, OMD may lead to trauma and damage of the structures of the oral cavity, dental restorations, and dentures. Thus, jaw-closing dystonia may result in excessive dental wear, dental fractures, and trauma of the lips, gums, and tongue, whereas jaw-opening dystonia may be associated with temporomandibular joint overload and dislocations. Consequently, there is need for both dental and neurological efforts as well as collaboration between the two professions, although the diagnosis is neurological.

To illustrate the diversity of oromandibular dystonia and the need for careful control of BoNT treatment, two patients are presented in the following section. First patient is a woman with focal oromandibular dystonia and blepharospasms. She was referred for examination 15 years earlier when she was 60 years. Her condition started 5 years previously in the eye region. Later chewing and swallowing problems arose. In addition, constant and strong biting and grinding movements developed, causing fractures of dental restorations and severe attrition of the teeth. She used a bite splint but her dentition was also challenged by her drug-induced hyposalivation that contributed to increased caries activity and dental erosions. Besides clonazepam for the dystonia, she was also medicated with psychoactive drugs and BoNT for the blepharospasms. She felt her dystonia as a severe handicap and therefore quit her job as secretary. Her dystonia changed over the 15 years (**Figure 4**). It grew worse also including the lips.

The BoNT/A injections were adjusted accordingly and were able to reduce the high spontaneous activity (**Figure 5**). In spite of the regular treatments, 3.3 BoNT series per year, the dentition deteriorated and was reduced from consisting of a full complement of 29 with only 3 wisdom tooth missing, to 5 remaining natural tooth and prosthetic restorations (**Figure 6**).

http://dx.doi.org/10.5772/64271

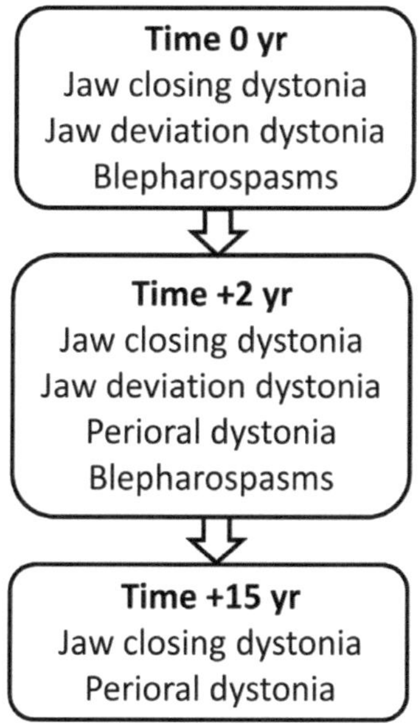

Figure 4. Shifts of dystonia types during a 15-year period in an elderly woman.

Time +10 yr Spontaneous activity (EMG µV) Muscles		Before A/Ona	Units A/Ona	2 months after A/Ona	Reference Values M±SD
Temporalis	R	24	20	8	3.5±1.9
	L	20	20	12	
Masseter	R	17	25	7	2.4±1.0
	L	9	25	5	
Medial pterygoid	R	20	15	6	11.5±4.5
	L	9	15	4	
Anterior digastric	R	44	0	22	4.0±2.5
	L	32	0	19	
Lateral pterygoid	R	12	25	8	11.0±4.5
	L	33	25	9	
Orbicularis oris superior	R	14	5	6	4.0±2.0
	L	15	5	5	
Orbicularis oris inferior	R	45	10	9	5.3±2.5
	L	34	10	5	

Figure 5. Electromyographic recordings of spontaneous muscle activity in an elderly woman with oromandibular dystonia immediately before and after a BoNT treatment series. The activity is clearly reduced from the treatment, even in the nontreated digastric muscles (bipolar surface electrodes, mean voltage; custom-designed eight-channel EMG system; Electromyographic Laboratory, Dept. of Odontology, University of Copenhagen).

Fifteen years after the diagnosis, the dystonia was reduced compared to previous years. There were fewer outbursts of dystonic activity and the involuntary jaw closing and lip dystonia was less powerful. In spite of her tooth loss, the patient was satisfied with her dentures and her chewing function had improved.

The second patient is a woman referred 17 years earlier when she was 59 years. She had gradually developed an anterior mandibular overjet through some months and could only with difficulty bite the teeth together with normal incisor relationships. There was no pain associated with the condition, but increasing chewing and speech problems. She was diagnosed with jaw deviation associated with dystonia of the lateral pterygoid muscle on both sides.

	Molars			Pre-molars		Canines	Incisors				Canines	Pre-molars		Molars		
Time 0 yr		7	6	5	4	3	2	1	1	2	3	4	5	6	7	
		7	6	5	4	3	2	1	1	2	3	4	5	6	7	8
	Molars			Pre-molars		Canines	Incisors				Canines	Pre-molars		Molars		
Time +2 yr			6		4	3	2	1	1	2	3	4		6	7	
			6	5	4	3	2		1	2	3	4	5			8
	Molars			Pre-molars		Canines	Incisors				Canines	Pre-molars		Molars		
Time +15 yr	Partial denture						2	1	1	2	3	Partial denture				
	Full denture															

Figure 6. Reduction in the number of teeth in an elderly woman during 15 years with oromandibular dystonia. The deterioration of the dentition was associated with fractures of dental restorations and severe attrition of the teeth from the dystonic jaw movements combined with increased caries activity and dental erosions from hyposalivation.

Her habitual occlusion was displaced 4–5 mm anteriorly to the normal sagittal relationship, a so-called mandibular overjet. However, analysis of the dental attrition on plaster models revealed that the original occlusion in the front was a 2-mm maxillary overjet, that is, a normal sagittal relationship between the maxillary and mandibular anterior teeth. In contrast to the patient with focal dystonia, the jaw deviation dystonia did not change over time. No other muscles were involved. At first, treatment the lateral pterygoid muscles were injected with 20 units A/Ona each, and later on with 40 units each (**Figure 7**). The type of dystonia was unchanged during 17 years in contrast to the female patient mentioned earlier. An excellent treatment effect was obtained with complete reversal of the jaw protrusion and normalization of chewing and speech, and it was repeated again and again with A/Ona injections on an average 1.7 times per year (**Figure 8**).

http://dx.doi.org/10.5772/64271

Time +3 yr Spontaneous activity (EMG µV) Muscles		Before A/Ona	Units A/Ona	2 months after A/Ona	Reference Values M±SD
Temporalis	R	4	0	3	3.5±1.9
	L	3	0	3	
Masseter	R	5	0	14	2.4±1.0
	L	4	0	9	
Anterior digastric	R	5	0	4	4.0±2.5
	L	6	0	5	
Lateral pterygoid	R	50	40	15	11.0±4.5
	L	38	40	5	

Figure 7. Electromyographic recordings of spontaneous muscle activity in an elderly woman with jaw deviation dystonia immediately before and after a BoNT treatment series. The injections in the lateral pterygoid muscles reduced the activity in the treated muscles and normalized the dental occlusion (bipolar electrodes, mean voltage; custom-designed 8-channel EMG system; Electromyographic Laboratory, Dept. of Odontology, University of Copenhagen).

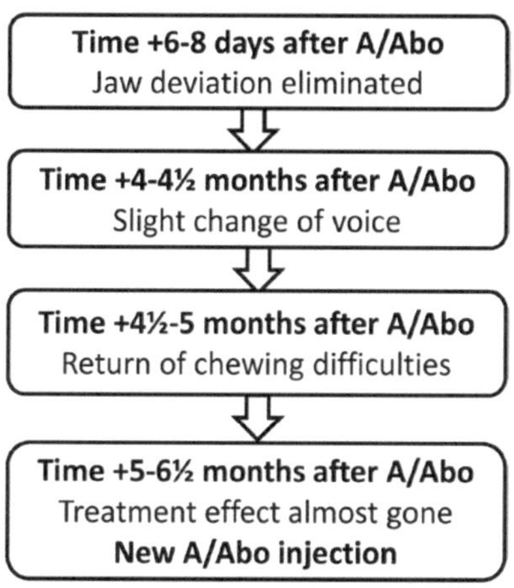

Figure 8. Unchanged jaw deviation dystonia persisting during a 17-year period in an elderly woman.

2.4. Special conditions

Besides the already mentioned conditions, BoNT may be helpful in special situations as a palliative intervention. Bite wounds in the tongue, lips, and cheeks may occur after accidental or involuntary jaw closures in patients with cerebral palsy, parkinsonian syndromes, dementia, or in retarded persons. Intramuscular injections with BoNT may attenuate bite force and thus reduce the possibility of severe lesions. Frequent dislocations of the temporomandibular joints represent a serious problem. They imply frequent contacts with the health care system and the emergency wards. Such habitual dislocations may result from neurological disorders, articular hypermobility, or sequelae after jaw trauma. BoNT injections into the lateral pterygoid muscle, in one or both sides, may reduce the problem if the situation is very frustrating and painful [21].

3. Drooling and secretory disorders of the salivary glands

Saliva secretion amounts to about 1 L per day with higher secretion rates during chewing and taste stimulation than at rest [22]. Under normal physiological conditions, the resting secretion rate of whole saliva is 0.2–0.5 ml per min during wakefulness and practically negligible during sleep. The most important salivary glands are the parotid and the submandibular glands. They have different functional patterns. Unstimulated the submandibular gland secretes the majority of the saliva. In the stimulated state, the saliva production from the parotid and the submandibular glands is approximately the same.

3.1. Drooling

Usually the saliva is swallowed unconsciously throughout the day. Unintentional loss of saliva from the mouth, referred to as sialorrhoea or drooling, is most often due to decreased swallowing function rather than regular hypersalivation [23]. Drooling is unusual after the age of 5 years. In adults it is often related to gastroesophageal reflux, pregnancy, or develops as a side effect of pharmacological treatment. Even patients with a low salivary flow rate may suffer from sialorrhoea, when impaired swallowing function leads to accumulation of saliva in mouth, and when insufficient lip closure or reduced oral sensitivity causes overflow and loss of saliva from the mouth. If the saliva passes over the lower lip, it may run down the chin and drip on the clothing, or it may be aspirated and cause coughing and lung inflammation. Thus, drooling both results in reduced quality of life and poses a significant health risk.

Severe and psychosocially embarrassing drooling occurs especially in congenital or acquired neurological disorders, such as parkinsonian syndromes, amyotrophic lateral sclerosis, and cerebral palsy. Therefore, the general diagnosis and treatment of this type of drooling are primarily within the working area for neurologists and takes place in a hospital setting. However, dentists must be able to identify the problem in order to refer for treatment. The treatment consists essentially in reducing the saliva secretion (**Figure 9**).

Such treatment may induce severe side effects in terms of dry mouth depending on its type, which range from irreversible surgical interventions and radiation to reversible treatments with intraglandular BoNT injections. As a consequence, the treatment may also cause accelerated caries progression and other oral disorders. To minimize or prevent such development, the patient should be followed closely by a dentist. However, as BoNT is one of the least invasive treatments for drooling, it should always be considered as a relevant option. Based on clinical evidence, treatment of severe drooling with percutaneous BoNT injections bilaterally into the parotid and submandibular glands is considered useful [25].

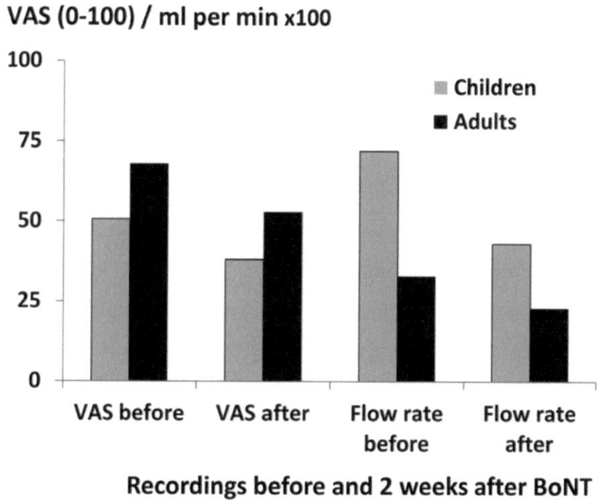

Figure 9. The effect of intraglandular injections into each parotid and submandibular gland with 15–40 units onabotulinumtoxinA (A/Ona) or incobotulinumtoxinA (A/Inco) evaluated by visual analog scales (VAS) for drooling discomfort and unstimulated whole saliva flow rate (ml/min × 100). Mean values before and 2 weeks after the treatment in 14 children with cerebral palsy and in 9 adults with amyotrophic lateral sclerosis and Parkinson's disease [2, 24].

Before the treatment start, it is important to record the frequency and extent of the drooling as well as the impact of the drooling problem. The unstimulated salivary secretion rate should be measured to clarify the cause and to determine the BoNT dose. Depending on the cooperation from the patient, saliva can be collected either in a cup by the draining method or by a modified swab method with dental cotton rolls. Intraglandular injections with BoNT should be given with ultrasonographic guidance to place the bolus centrally in the glands to ensure maximum efficiency and minimize the side effects (**Figure 10**) [2, 24].

Light anesthesia or sedation may be necessary, especially in children, because the injections are associated with local discomfort or pain and therefore provoke avert reaction and movements. Most clinical reports include treatments with commercially available preparations of type BoNT/A, such as A/Ona and A/Inco, with 15–40 units in each parotid gland and in each submandibular gland. Compositions of BoNT/B such as B/Rima in doses of 750–2500 units have also been used for drooling, for example, Møller et al. [1]. The treatment effect of BoNT is local. It has few side effects, which is usually short lasting and results from the injection trauma. In few cases, there may be difficulty in swallowing due to impaired muscle activity usually lasting some weeks. In all circumstances, the effect is temporary, and largely gone after 3 months. Repetition of the treatment and possible dose modifications should depend on the effect of treatment, the current secretions rate, the drooling level, and the extent of any adverse effects.

In children and young subjects, spontaneous cessation of drooling may occur as a result of the physiological development [2]. Therefore, the drooling treatment should not be performed automatically. It must be ensured that the drooling problems have returned after the expected duration of the treatment effect before performing a new treatment. As a consequence, it is advisable that treatment of drooling in these age groups is reversible, such as intraglandular injections with BoNT, as more invasive types of treatment with long-term or permanent effect [2].

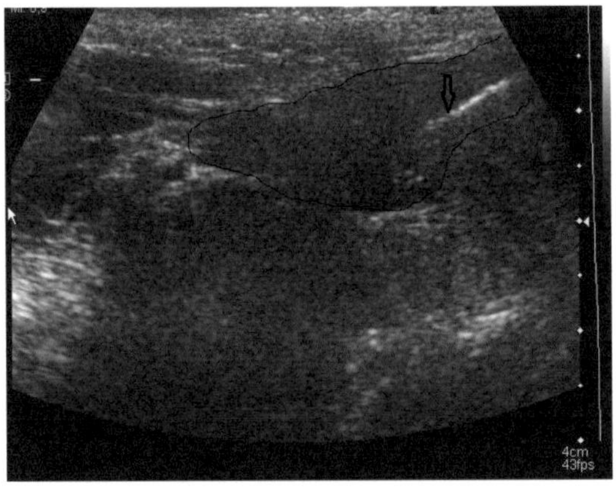

Figure 10. Ultrasonographic guidance during intraglandular injection of BoNT into the submandibular gland. The tip of the injection needle is indicated by an arrow. (GE Logiq 9, "thyroid" settings; 12 MHz linear transducer).

3.2. Frey's syndrome

Frey's syndrome or gustatory sweating in the preauricular area is an unpleasant phenomenon typically appearing during meals. It may also be socially disabling when flushing and intense sweating with subsequent wetting of clothes prevents the patient from eating in company. The syndrome occurs after surgical procedures or traumas on the parotid gland. Frey's syndrome is most likely caused by misdirected regeneration of cut or damaged parasympathetic fibers, producing new "salivary" reflex arches activating sweat glands and small subcutaneous blood vessels instead of salivary gland tissue. Thus, sweating and vasodilatation appear in the reinnervated area when salivation is induced upon cholinergic stimulation from gustatory and masticatory stimuli [26]. Intradermal injections of BoNT/A may be considered for gustatory sweating and seems clinically effective [27]. It has also been suggested that Frey's syndrome should be viewed as a dynamic process in which the stimulus for aberrant reinnervation of parasympathetic nerve fibers can be reduced in some patients, with BoNT injections to the treated areas [28]. Thus, the gustatory sweating may fade over time and does not necessarily have to be retreated over and over again.

To localize the extent of involved skin area, Minor's iodine-starch test is used before treatment. An iodine solution (castor oil mixed with 2% iodine alcohol solution 1:9) is applied on the skin of the involved cheek and dried for 0.5 min, and potato flour is spread out evenly and thinly through a sieve over the area. During chewing of slices of apple, or sucking sour or strong-flavored candies for 5 min, a chemical reaction takes place between iodine and starch. This leaves the zones of perspiration dark brown. Then the surplus of flour is gently removed by compressed air and suction (**Figure 11**).

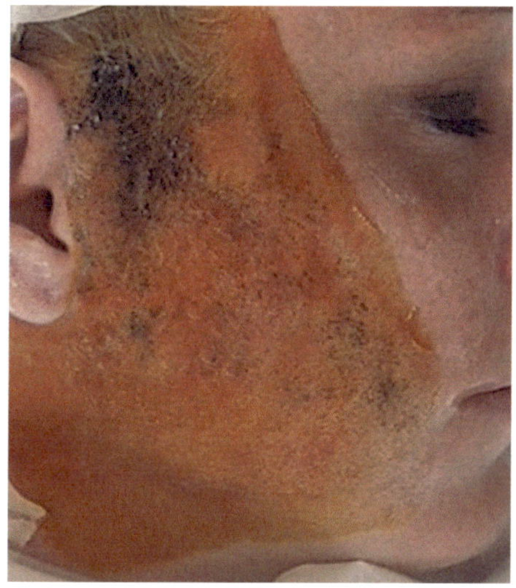

Figure 11. Frey's syndrome or gustatory sweating after stabbing of the face in a 37-year-old woman. Dark brown spotted areas with perspiration obtained by the Minor's iodine-starch test after eating apple.

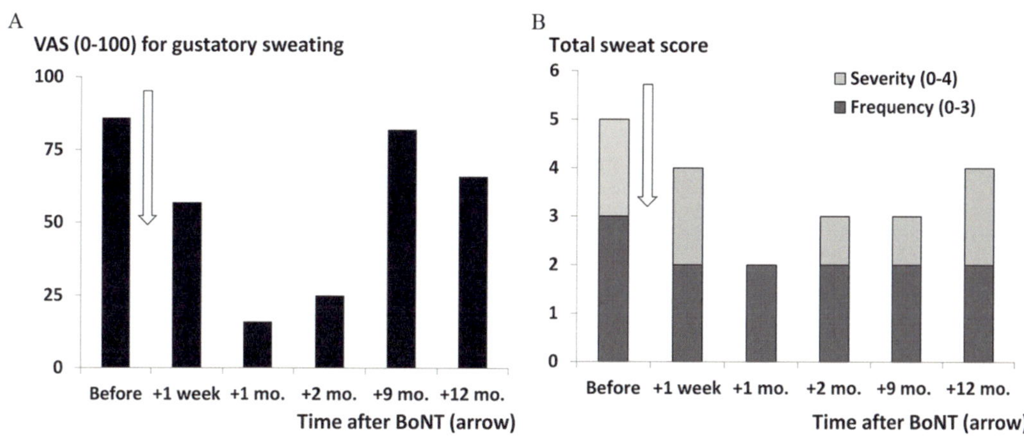

Figure 12. Frey's syndrome or gustatory sweating after stabbing of the face in a 37-year-old woman. A: Self-reported impact of discomfort and problems with perspiration of the cheek in daily life on horizontal visual analog scales (VAS) before treatment and at follow-ups during 1 year after treatment. B: Self-reported total score for severity and frequency of gustatory sweating (0–7) before treatment and at follow-ups during 1 year after treatment (modified after Thomas-Stonell and Greenberg [29]).

The distribution of the zones can be documented using a digital camera and by evaluating the skin areas morphometrically [28]. The distribution of the dark brown spotted areas may also be transferred to an acetate template with anatomical landmarks corresponding to ear, eye, and mouth for reference during the injections [26]. Local anesthetic cream is applied to the involved skin areas before BoNT treatment as the repeated intradermal injections may be rather painful. The injections are made at 1-cm distances, that is, one single injection per

1 cm^2, and for each injection, 0.5 units A/Ona or A/Inco is used [26]. After about 1 week, the perspiration is reduced (**Figure 12A** and **B**), especially the severity. After treatment, not only the sweating is reduced. The treated areas may also remain pale when the cheeks otherwise blush during physical exercise or fitness. The effect may last for 0.5–1 year.

4. Conclusion

Several conditions in the oromandibular region may benefit from treatment with BoNT injections. The treatment is local, and there are few side effects if the injections are guided by electromyography and/or ultrasonography. However, animal studies indicate that changes in muscle fibers and bone loss may be a risk factor for the use of BoNT in jaw muscles [30, 31]. In any circumstances, the treatment should be planned by thorough examination of possible injection targets, and the effect of the treatments must be controlled. The dose and targets should not be repeated routinely but must be adjusted in repeated injection series based on analysis of the effect. To get the best results and minimize or prevent side effects, collaboration between doctors with several different professional backgrounds is important.

Author details

Merete Bakke[1*], Torben Dalager[2] and Eigild Møller[2]

*Address all correspondence to: mbak@sund.ku.dk

1 Department of Odontology, Faculty of Health and Medical Sciences, University of Copenhagen, Copenhagen, Denmark

2 Department of Neurology, Bispebjerg University Hospital, University of Copenhagen, Copenhagen, Denmark

References

[1] Møller E, Daugaard D, Holm O, Winge K, Bardow A, Lykkeaa J, Belhage B, Bakke M. Repeated treatments of drooling with botulinum toxin B in neurology. Acta Neurol Scand. 2015;131: 51–57.

[2] Møller E, Pedersen SA, Vinicoff PG, Bardow A, Svendsen P, Bakke M. Onabotulinum A treatment of drooling in children with cerebral palsy: a prospective, longitudinal open-label study. Toxins (Basel). 2015;7: 2481–2493.

[3] Møller E, Bakke M, Dalager T, Werdelin LM. Oromandibular dystonia involving the lateral pterygoid muscles: four cases with different complexity. Mov Disord. 2007;22:785–790.

[4] Fuglsang-Frederiksen A, Ostergaard L, Sjö O, Werdelin L, Winkel H. Quantitative electromyographical changes in cervical dystonia after treatment with botulinum toxin. Electromyogr Clin Neurophysiol. 1998;38:75–79.

[5] Bakke M, Werdelin LM, Dalager T, Fuglsang-Frederiksen A, Prytz S, Møller E. Reduced jaw opening from paradoxical activity of mandibular elevator muscles treated with botulinum toxin. Eur J Neurol. 2003;10:695–699.

[6] Møller E, Werdelin LM, Bakke M, Dalager T, Prytz S, Regeur L. Treatment of perioral dystonia with botulinum toxin in 4 cases of Meige's syndrome. Oral Surg Oral Med Oral Pathol Oral Radiol Endod. 2003;96:544–549.

[7] Yun JY, Kim JW, Kim HT, Chung SJ, Kim JM, Cho JW, Lee JY, Lee HN, You S, Oh E, Jeong H, Kim YE, Kim HJ, Lee WY, Jeon BS. Dysport and Botox at a ratio of 2.5:1 units in cervical dystonia: a double-blind, randomized study. Mov Disord. 2015;30:206–213.

[8] Rosales RL, Ng AR, Santos MM, Fernandez HH. The broadening application of chemodenervation in X-linked dystonia-parkinsonism (Part II): an open-label experience with botulinum toxin-A (Dysport®) injections for oromandibular, lingual, and truncal-axial dystonias. Int J Neurosci. 2011;121 Suppl 1:44–56.

[9] Møller E. The chewing apparatus. An electromyographic study of the action of the muscles of mastication and its correlation to facial morphology., Acta Physiol Scand Suppl. 1966;280:1–229.

[10] Prevalence of TMJD and its signs and symptoms [Internet]. Available from: htp://www.nidrcr.nih.gov/DataStatistics/FindDataByTopic/FacialPain/PrevalenceTMJD.htm [Accessed: 2016-4-1].

[11] Greene CS, American Association for Dental Research. Diagnosis and treatment of temporomandibular disorders: emergence of a new care guidelines statement. Oral Surg Oral Med Oral Pathol Oral Radiol Endod. 2010;110:137–139.

[12] Ernberg M, Hedenberg-Magnusson B, List T et al. Efficacy of botulinum toxin type A for treatment of persistent myofascial TMD pain: a randomized, controlled, double-blind multicenter study. Pain. 2011;152:1988–1996.

[13] Linde M, Hagen K, Stovner LJ. Botulinum toxin treatment of secondary headaches and cranial neuralgias: a review of evidence. Acta Neurol Scand. Suppl. 2011;191:50–55.

[14] Smyth AG. Botulinum toxin treatment of bilateral masseteric hypertrophy. Br J Oral Maxillofac Surg. 1994;32:29–33.

[15] Moore AP, Wood GD. The medical management of masseteric hypertrophy with botulinum toxin type A. Br J Oral Maxillofac Surg. 1994;32:26–28.

[16] Fedorowics Z, van Zuuren EJ, Schoones J. Botulinum toxin for masseter hypertrophy. Cochrane Database Syst Rev. 2013;9:CD007510.

[17] Bakke M, Holm B, Jensen BL, Michler L, Møller E. Unilateral, isometric bite force in 8-68-year-old women and men related to occlusal factors. Scand J Dent Res. 1990;98:149–158.

[18] Bakke M, Møller E, Thomsen CE, Dalager T, Werdelin LM. Chewing in patients with severe neurological impairment. Arch Oral Biol. 2007;52:399–403.

[19] Bakke M, Larsen BM, Dalager T, Møller E. Oromandibular dystonia–functional and clinical characteristics: a report on 21 cases. Oral Surg Oral Med Oral Pathol Oral Radiol. 2013;115:e21–26.

[20] Møller E, Bakke M, Dalager T, Werdelin LM, Lonsdale MN, Højgaard L, Friberg L. Somatosensory input and oromandibular dystonia. Clin Neurol Neurosurg. 2013;115:1141–1143.

[21] Fu KY, Chen HM, Sun ZP, Zhang ZK, Ma XC. Long-term efficacy of botulinum toxin type A for the treatment of habitual dislocation of the temporomandibular joint. Br J Oral Maxillofac Surg. 2010;48:281–284.

[22] Sreebny LM. Saliva in health and disease: an appraisal and update. Int Dent J. 2000;50:140–161.

[23] Bakke M, Bardow A, Møller E. Severe drooling and treatment with botulinum toxin. ASHA SIG 13 Perspectives on Swallowing and Swallowing Disorders (Dysphagia). 2012;21:15–21.

[24] Møller E, Karlsborg M, Bardow A, Lykkeaa J, Nissen FH, Bakke M. Treatment of severe drooling with botulinum toxin in amyotrophic lateral sclerosis and Parkinsons's disease: efficacy and possible mechanisms. Acta Odontol Scand 2011;69:151–157.

[25] Naumann M, So Y, Argoff CE, Childers MK, Dykstra DD, Gronseth GS, Jabbari B, Kaufmann HC, Schurch B, Silberstein SD, Simpson DM; Therapeutics and Technology Assessment Subcommittee of the American Academy of Neurology. Assessment: botulinum neurotoxin in the treatment of autonomic disorders and pain (an evidence-based review): report of the Therapeutics and Technology Assessment Subcommittee of the American Academy of Neurology. Neurology 2008;70:1707–1714.

[26] Bakke M, Max Thorsen N, Bardow A, Dalager T, Eckhart Thomsen C, Regeur L. Treatment of gustatory sweating with low-dose botulinum toxin A: a case report. Acta Odontol Scand. 2006;64:129–133.

[27] Steffen A, Rotter N, König IR, Wollenberg B. Botulinum toxin for Frey's syndrome: a closer look at different treatment responses. J Laryngol Otol. 2012;126:185–189.

[28] Eckardt A, Kuettner C. Treatment of gustatory sweating (Frey's syndrome) with botulinum toxin A. Head Neck. 2003;25:624–628.

http://dx.doi.org/10.5772/64271

[29] Thomas-Stonell N, Greenberg J. Three treatment approaches and clinical factors in the reduction of drooling. Dysphagia. 1988;3:73–78.

[30] Korfage JAM, Wang J, Langenbach GEJ. Influence of botulinum toxin on rabbit jaw muscle activity and anatomy. Muscle Nerve. 2012;45:684–691.

[31] Matthys T, Dang HAH, Rafferty KL, Herring SW. Bone and cartilage changes in rabbit mandibular condyles after 1 injection of botulinum toxin. Am J Orthod Dentofacial Orthop. 2015;148:999–1009.

Chapter 8

How Does Botulinum Toxin Injection and Physiotherapy Complement Each Other in Cerebral Palsy?

Ayşe Numanoğlu Akbaş

Additional information is available at the end of the chapter

http://dx.doi.org/10.5772/66693

Abstract

Cerebral Palsy (CP) is a clinical condition that describes impairments of motor and sensory systems due to a lesion in immature brain. CP-related disorders effect movements, balance and posture of the child. Spasticity is most frequent motor disorder seen in CP and effects 70–80% of the children with CP. Spasticity can lead to abnormalities in all motor system levels involving muscles, joints, bones and tendons. If spasticity exists for long period of time, immobilization of muscles in short position and changes in the connective tissue around joints lead to shortening of the muscles and connective tissue. Various methods are used for spasticity management in children with CP. Botulinum neurotoxin (BoNT) injections, oral medications, selective dorsal rhizotomy and intrathecal baclofen applications are the foremost among them. BoNT injections are most prevalently used one among these applications. BoNT, which is a neurotoxin obtained from *Clostridium botulinum* bacteria, is frequently used in children with CP to decrease muscle tone for a certain period in the selected muscles, prevent contractures, postpone surgery and decrease frequency of surgeries. During this time frame that muscle tone decreased, it is very important to increase activity and participation levels of children. For achieving better motor outcomes and functional independence, BoNT injections should be combined with physiotherapy (PT) and occupational therapy (OT).

Keywords: botulinum toxin, cerebral palsy, physiotherapy, spasticity, occupational therapy

1. Introduction

BoNT/A injections are one of the most frequently used methods to reduce muscle tone in individuals with CP. Given with clinical precision, BoNT/A has reversible chemo-denervation effects, such that focal applications in selected muscles ensure selective muscle relaxation to intended muscles. BoNT/A was used in CP for the first time in 1993 by Koman et al. [1]. It has been used in gradually increasing rates since the day it was first used and in wider age ranges. The purpose of this section is to explain how BoNT injections and physiotherapy (PT) approaches complement each other. In this section, general information about CP, changes that occur in muscles due to spasticity, outcome measurements related with BoNT/A applications, combined usage of BoNT/A applications with PT and occupational therapy (OT) approaches, target muscles for injection, appropriate age range and side effects of injections will be discussed.

2. Cerebral palsy definition and classification

Cerebral palsy (CP) defines a group of permanent disorders of movement and posture development that causes activity limitation; these disorders are related with nonprogressive influence, lesion or anomalies that occur in developing brain. Disorders of communication and behavior, sensation, perceptional, cognitional problems and epilepsy generally accompany motor disorders of CP [2, 3]. These disorders affect body movements, balance and posture negatively [4–6].

Surveillance of Cerebral Palsy in Europe (SCPE) [2] classifies CP as spastic, dyskinetic and ataxic type based on the predominant neurologic findings. Majority (70–80%) of children with CP have spastic clinic characteristics. Increased muscle tone of the effected extremities, increased deep tendon reflexes, muscular weakness, tremor, abnormal posture and movement patterns, increased coactivation of antagonistic muscles, abnormal control of voluntary movement and associated movements and stereotypical movements are seen in spastic type [7–9].

Classification of children with CP according to anatomic pattern and special neuromotor effect is crucial for the treatment of motor disorders [10]. The most important major classification in children with CP is the classification made according to the anatomic pattern of effect. Hemiparesis, where only half of the body is affected; diparesis, where lower extremities are affected basically and upper extremities are affected slightly; and quadriparesis, where all extremities are affected, are the most widespread definitions [10]. In recent years, the idea suggested by SCPE for the spastic type has started to be accepted for CP classification; as "unilateral spastic CP" where a single side of the body is affected or "bilateral spastic CP" where both sides are affected [2].

3. Spasticity

Spasticity, widely seen in CP, is the increase of physiologic muscle tone. Spasticity can occur in different forms depending on the formation time, location, size and diffuseness of the lesion in the developing central nervous system [11].

Fibrous contractures inside muscle or connective tissue around joints originating from spastic extremity posture, which are forming over time, compromise the increased response of the muscle against passive stretch and are one of the reasons of increased muscle tone. Muscle contractures and spasticity generally complicate patient care and reduce extremity functions and motor capacity [11–13].

CP is caused by nonprogressive lesion in the brain but accompanying spasticity, reduced muscle strength, muscle length changes, abnormalities in joint movements, functional capacity deficiencies and many situations like this are not static and can change over time with growth. Musculoskeletal system pathologies may start to cause greater problems as child grows. For normal muscle growth, elongation of the muscle under physiological overload is necessary. A hypertonic muscle, unable to relax, will eventually fail to grow and develop with the normal elongation of the bone in a child. Increase in height and weight of the child can contribute to musculoskeletal system problems. Spasticity can cause contractures and torsional deformities due to the growth in bones and muscles not being in proportion. Moreover, instability and early osteoarthritic changes can be observed in joints. As the individuals with CP grow, abnormal biomechanical situations affecting joints and static postures can cause pain formation. As the child grows old, chronic pain, social isolation, functional limitations and dependency can affect mental status negatively [7, 14].

4. Tone inhibition in children with CP

BoNT/A injections relax muscles by blocking acetylcholine release, with pharmacologic effect occurring in 48–72 h, but which wanes 3–4 months later [7]. However, this period when tone decreases gives an opportunity for therapeutic approaches [7, 15]. BoNT/A injections in children with CP are generally combined with PT and OT, while trying to achieve better rehabilitation outcomes. This complementary application has been accepted generally because it can be applied to the spastic muscles directly and the amount of the toxin can be adjusted per muscle, and it has rapid effect and has only a few side effects [16, 17]. But tone reduction alone is not enough for gaining functional outcomes. Applications such as stretching and strengthening the muscles, weight bearing on extremities and practicing daily life activities are essential. Children need to continue an intensive physiotherapy program before and after the BoNT/A application for achieving functional improvements [18].

Many studies investigate to maximize this effect of BoNT/A injections. In this perspective, combined usage of PT and BoNT/A has been discussed. This temporary effect of BoNT/A can be increased by activity-based physiotherapy and rehabilitation programs [15]. The decrease of tone by selective chemodenervation of overactive muscles presents an opportunity to extend muscle length, prevent contracture formation, strengthen antagonistic muscles, introduce new movement strategies to children and improve motor and functional skills [19, 20].

It was reported that PT and OT approaches that are used in children with CP in combination with BoNT/A injections are conventional PT, conventional OT, constrained induced movement therapy (CIMT), hand-arm bimanual intensive training (HABIT), casting, active/passive stretching exercises, strengthening exercises, neurodevelopmental approach (Bobath), robotic rehabilitation and mobility and walking training [15, 21–25].

Although the benefits of BoNT/A injections with PT and OT combinations are mentioned in many studies, optimal intensity and dosage of the therapies to be applied is not known [16]. According to expert opinion and consensus reports, PT following BoNT/A injections must consist of functional motor training, serial casting, stretching and strengthening exercises [26–28]. According to the literature, PT and OT programs can be followed-up as individualized therapy, group therapy, distance learning or a home program by family education [29–31].

5. Classification in CP

Classification systems have been developed to determine the severity of functional limitations in CP. The most important and widely used one of these systems is the Gross Motor Function Classification System (GMFCS) developed by Palisano et al. (1997). This system comprises five levels: level I expresses the best level of gross motor function and level V expresses the most influence in motor function. According to this system, the children in level I can walk independently, and the children in level V cannot sit independently without a support and cannot protect their head and body postures against gravity [32].

It is reported that BoNT/A application is used generally in ambulant hemiplegic and diplegic children with mild or moderate motor influence. The reason for an increase usage in this population depends on the acquisition of greater functional gains of these children [33]. In mildly affected children, tone of the spastic, active and nonfibrotic muscles can be decreased until 12–16 weeks [27, 34, 35]. In children with severe motor disorders, on the other hand, this gain is more limited. In children who are at GMFCS level 4–5, even very simple tasks used in daily life could generate problems and affect quality of life negatively [36, 37]. Although BoNT/A injections are used in these children to facilitate active movement, to ease their care and to decrease pain, there are not adequate evidences reporting the effect of these applications [33].

Researchers report that small children with CP at GMFCS level I–II show better development in gross motor function, on the other hand, older children in GMFCS level III–IV show less development in gross motor function or no development at all. The possibility of development of contractures in older children with worse gross motor function level diminishes benefiting possibility from BoNT/A injection. Especially in GMFCS level IV–V children, dysphagia, respiration problems, brain stem pathology and cranial nerve influence accompany more and therefore it is reported that BoNT/A dose for these children must be adjusted very carefully [27, 34].

6. Physiotherapy and occupational therapy approaches frequently used in CP

The purpose of therapy in CP is to improve functionality, support skill development and locomotion, sustain health in terms of social interaction and independency and to prevent possible deformities. Best results are achieved by early intense intervention. For an effective treatment program, team approach including physiotherapy, occupational therapy, behavioral therapy, pharmacological and surgical treatment, adaptive equipment and therapy and treatment of related health problems is necessary. The purpose of all treatment methods is to improve independency of the child [7, 10].

PT and OT applications start at birth and continue through life span to minimize sensory and motor disorders, to support normal motor development of the children, to improve activity and participation, to facilitate activities of daily life and to reduce load of family and caretakers. However, increased muscle tone, whose negative effects were mentioned in detail above, complicates physiotherapy and OT applications and is shown as one of the reasons of unresponsiveness to PT in children with CP [19]. Therefore, PT and OT approaches must be combined with applications helping tone control such as BoNT/A injections. Most frequently used physiotherapy approaches in children with CP are neurodevelopmental treatment (Bobath); based on normal sense-motor development of children, Vojta; using reflex stimulus points, Avres; suggesting that sensory-motor integration and organization is the basic of psychomotor development and conductive education (Peto), where intensive training programs are applied in the management by a leader and Goal Directed Therapy determining individual targets [18]. Numerous different therapy methods including electrotherapy applications, muscle strengthening and stretching exercises, orthotics, adaptive equipment and serial casting can also be used along with these approaches.

7. Evidences on physiotherapy approaches in combination with BoNT/A injections

BoNT/A injection in CP is considered as a selective tool to reduce spasticity. Appropriate selection of the patient, treatment dosage and muscles is crucial for effective injections [19]. In the scope of the International Classification and Functioning (ICF), BoNT/A injections affect body structures and functions; however, when it is combined with physiotherapy, it causes changes in the activity level as well [16]. The effectiveness of physiotherapy programs changes based on the application period and intensity [15]. Moreover, experience and knowledge level of physiotherapist, context of home program and conformity of the families to home program is crucial for the effectiveness of the treatment. There is no consensus on the type of exercises, or rehabilitation methods should be used to maximize the effects of tone reduction following BoNT/A applications. It is reported that orthotic management, serial casting and intensive physiotherapy are the most significant factors to benefit the most from the injection effect [19, 38].

It is reported that age of the patient, therapy applications and casting are crucial factors improving success following BoNT/A injections [39]. Inclusion of especially strengthening exercises and targeted motor training within the physiotherapy program is suggested [27].

The effects of PT + BoNT/A injections are reported as the reduction in spasticity, increase in dynamic and passive range of motion, improvement in selective motor control, improvement in strength, improvement in function and task performance and reduction in pain [27].

There are numerous studies in the literature investigating the usage of PT and BoNT/A applications together. In a study, the effectiveness of BoNT/A injections in long term with and without physiotherapy was determined. One of the groups received regular PT (two times a week) while other group received intensive PT. It was reported that gross motor function showed more improvement in the intensive PT group at the end of 1 year. Although tone increased after a period, gross motor function scores were preserved. It has been emphasized that BoNT/A injections decreased muscle tone in children with CP and when combined with PT the benefits of this application improved (Jianjun, Shurong et al. 2013).

In a study comparing the influence the two different PT methods, an intense physiotherapy program consisting of NDT (focusing on motor development and function) was applied to a group while conventional intense physiotherapy program (focusing on muscle length and strength) was applied in the other group. It was reported that the children benefited from both interventions; however, the success in NDT group was higher in terms of reaching the determined targets [19].

Chaturvedi et al. compared two groups of children with CP; one group received PT and other group received PT + BoNT/A injection. After 6 months of rehabilitation, they reported that gross motor function improved in both groups and also there was increase in the sensory and motor fiber diameter measured by diffusion tensor tractography; in other words, brain plasticity improved. They discussed that BoNT/A injections made as an addition to PT did not affect the result in 6 months [15].

Improvement of hip abduction angle, popliteal angle and passive dorsal flexion was reported in individuals who received intense physiotherapy including use of ankle foot orthosis (AFO) after BoNT/A application [40]. In a research conducted on 29 children with CP and spastic equinus deformity, it was reported that tone reduction and dorsal flexion improvement was good in cases which were applied BoNT + PT and serial casting and their effects were preserved in the long terms in comparison to the cases which were applied only BoNT + PT. However, in this study, PT program only includes stretching for ankle. Lack of an extensive physiotherapy program may have affected the results. In this study, the authors reported the pressure ulcers in three patients as negative effects of casting and failure to do exercise when casting was made was reported to be a disadvantage. They suggested to apply weight-bearing and isometric exercises during the casting period [41].

In a study measuring muscle activation patterns with surface electromyography (sEMG) after BoNT/A application combined with intensive PT, it was reported that this combination had positive effects on walking kinematics but had no effect on muscle activation patterns [42].

In 47 children with spastic CP who were applied PT (stretching of flexor muscles, strengthening extensor muscles, functional mobility training) for 12 weeks following multilevel BoNT/A injections for lower extremity muscles, it was reported that gross motor function measured by Gross Motor Function Measurement (GMFM) improved, and this improvement was preserved up to 1 year; however, there was no change in energy consumption [38].

PT applied in 71 children with CP consists of stretching of flexor muscles, balance training and walking training (five times a week in the first 3 weeks and three times a week during the following 8 weeks); along with multilevel BoNT/A injections at the lower extremities, it was reported that the muscle tone decreased in the follow-up in the first 3 months; however, this was not preserved in the follow-up in the 6 months and the improvement in gross motor function that was measured by GMFM was sustained in both 3 and 6 months [43].

According to a review conducted in 2009, it was reported that BoNT/A is an effective application for decreasing spasticity and functional improvements can be achieved with time limitation. However, the follow-up periods were up to 6–24 weeks in many studies and this made it difficult to determine long-term effects and the effects of the repeating injections [44]. In contradicting with the former review we mentioned, in a systematic review conducted in 2011, BoNT/A injections made separately or in combination with casting were not suggested; it has been discussed that there is not adequate evidence on the combinations of BoNT/A injections with PT and usual care [45].

In researches where BoNT/A injections are applied along with PT, failure to explain adequately the content and period of the applied physiotherapy approaches, which modalities were used and who performed the PT applications makes it difficult to select the most correct therapy approach to be combined with BoNT/A injections. Methodological differences can explain the different results obtained in these studies. However, as proven in the above given studies, it is observed that the integration of the two applications resulted with especially improvement in gross motor function in children with spastic CP.

8. Evidences on occupational therapy approaches in combination with BoNT/A injections

The greatest problem faced when working with children with unilateral spastic CP is the rehabilitation of paretic upper extremities. These children manage to stand up and walk more easily and spontaneously in general. Numerous different reasons such as spasticity, shortness and weakness of upper extremity muscles, limited joint movement, rotational deformities in the forearm and wrist bones, decreased unilateral skills, inadequate motor control and sensory problems affect functional development of the affected extremity in children with unilateral CP [46].

CIMT aiming to facilitate intense usage of the affected extremity and limiting the healthy extremity usage; HABIT facilitating combined usage of both extremities, and Goal Directed Therapy, determining individual targets have been reported during the recent years as evidence-based applications improving upper extremity activities following BoNT/A injections [47–49].

The purpose of the post injection therapy is to ensure motivation and new experiences and form an environment where the children can use their affected arm [50]. There are studies reporting that usage of the affected upper extremity in children with unilateral CP does not improve when BoNT /A injections are made separately without combining with the therapy [51].

In a study comparing the two groups who were applied modified CIMT and OT approach supporting bimanual activity following BoNT/A injections in children with unilateral CP, improvement was achieved in upper extremity performance, functional skills, occupational performance and goal attainment, and the groups were not superior to one another. Therefore, it is suggested that clinicians divert to specific goals and select the family friendly and comfortable application [52].

In a randomized controlled study, a group which was applied OT following BoNT/A injection and another group which was only applied OT was compared, and it was reported that more successful result in terms of bimanual performance was obtained in the group which was applied OT in combination with BoNT/A. The authors reported that there was improvement in terms of activated range of motion and goal performance in both the groups. However, they reported that in the ICF framework, the improvement in each domain was observed only in the group applied OT after BoNT/A injection [53].

According to a Cochrane systematic review published in 2010, it was emphasized that BoNT/A injection combined with OT in children with CP and having unilateral influence was more effective in reducing the disorder and improving activity level in comparison to only OT [51].

9. Appropriate muscle selection in CP

Existing pathologies of the children are considered for the selection of the muscles to be injected, and generally BoNT/A injection need to be made for more than one muscle at the same time in general to obtain change in walking and other functional activities [34, 54]. BoNT/A injections are applied most frequently for equinus and equinovarus deformities, knee and hip flexion spasticity, adductor spasticity and spasticity of the upper extremity (e.g. finger flexion, wrist flexion, ulnar deviation, elbow flexion and shoulder adduction injection). In ambulant children with CP, generally walking pathologies are considered for the selection of the muscles to be injected. In children those who have spastic equinus, injections are made mostly to gastrocnemius and soleus muscles; in those who have jump gait to gastrocnemius, soleus and hamstring muscles; in those who have scissoring and jump gait to gastrocnemius, soleus, hamstrings and adductor muscles; in those who have scissoring to hamstrings and adductor muscles; in those who have spastic knee flexion to hamstrings and in those who have only scissoring to adductor muscles [15, 22, 35, 55].

The reason for more frequent usage of BoNT/A injections in lower extremities is explained as containing fewer fine skills, improving movement and gaining better functionality to the children during their daily life activities [33]. Complexity of neural motor control during upper extremity functions limits the usage of BoNT/A injections in upper extremities [56].

10. Evaluation in CP

Various assessment methods are used in CP to evaluate combined effects of PT, OT and BoNT/A applications. Tone assessments are the major ones among these. There are various clinic scales, biomechanical evaluation tools and neurophysiologic evaluation methods to

ICF domain	Assessment tool
Body structures and function	Active and Passive ROM Ashworth/Modified Ashworth Scale Dynamic Sonoelastography Electromyography Goal Attainment Scale (GAS) Gross Motor Function Measurement (GMFM) Manuel Muscle Testing The Quality of Upper Extremity Skills Test (QUEST) Physician's Rating Scale (PRS) Selective Motor Control Assessment Tardieu/Modified Tardieu Scale Three-Dimensional Gait Analyses Visual Analogue Scale (VAS) WeeFIM_ (Functional Independence Measure)
Activity/participation	Gross Motor Function Measurement (GMFM) *Assisting Hand* Assessment (AHA) ABILHAND-Kids Questionnaire Bimanual Fine Motor Function (BFMF) Child Health Questionnaire (CHQ) Edinburgh Visual Gait Score (EVGS) Energy Expenditure Measures Goal Attainment Scale (GAS) Manual Ability Classification System (MACS) Observational Gait Scale Physician's Rating Scale (PRS) Six-Minute Walk Test The Quality of Upper Extremity Skills Test (QUEST) The *Canadian Occupational Performance Measure* (COPM) Three-Dimensional Gait Analyses Visual Analogue Scale (VAS) WeeFIM_ (Functional Independence Measure)
External/personal factors	*Goal Attainment Scaling* (GAS)

Table 1. Outcome measurements used in children with CP to assess effects of BoNT/A injections.

evaluate spasticity; however, there is no consensus about how spasticity can be evaluated the best. The most frequently used clinical scales are Ashworth/Modified Ashworth and Tardieu/Modified Tardieu scales [57, 58]. However, reliability of these scales is questioned. In a study, it was reported that for assessing medial hamstrings spasticity, MTS and MAS were less sensitive in comparison to the sEMG in the determination of changes following BoNT/A injection [59].

In addition, there are scales such as Spasticity Grading, Modified Composite Spasticity Index, Duncan Ely Test, New York University Tone Scale and the Hypertonia Assessment Tool (HAT) [60–62]. As biomechanical evaluation tools, myotonometer, sensors, Wartenberg Pendulum Test, dynamometer, goniometric measurement and robot supported evaluation tools are used [61, 63–67]. Electromyography, tonic stretch test and soleus muscle Hoffmann reflex (H-reflex) are neurophysiologic evaluation methods that could be used in spasticity evaluation [61, 68, 69].

In addition to spasticity, changes in muscle length, normal motor development and functions are also evaluated. According to the literature, the most frequently used measurement tools in this respect are Gross Motor Function Measure evaluating gross motor function, Three-Dimensional Gait Analyses, Six-Minute Walk Test and Physician's Rating Scale (PRS) evaluating walking parameters, electromyography evaluating muscle activations, dynamic sonoelastography evaluating intrinsic characteristics of muscles, *Assisting Hand* Assessment (AHA), The *Canadian Occupational Performance Measure* and The Quality of Upper Extremity Skills Test evaluating upper extremity functions, *Goal Attainment Scaling* evaluating the level of reaching the determined targets and The Pediatric Evaluation of Disability Inventory measuring functional independency. Also active and passive range of motion, selective motor control and manual muscle strength measurement are in use for this population. The distribution of the measurement tools that are used most frequently in publications based on ICF dimensions is shown in **Table 1** [17, 19, 24, 25, 34, 38, 49, 52, 53, 55, 70–75].

11. Changes occurring in the intrinsic structure of muscle with BoNT/A injection

It was reported that increased stretch reflex response of spasticity had both neural and nonneural components. Motor unit and reflex activity formed against muscle length growth is indicated as the neural foundation, and mental status, stress, fatigue, decreased sarcomere number and decreased flexibility, muscle stiffness and high collagen content in spastic muscle are indicated as the nonneural components [76, 77].

Positive effects targeted with BoNT/A injections on neural characteristics of muscles and therapy targeted on passive and active characteristics; therefore, combinations of these applications are suggested [33].

In a child with spastic diparetic CP, it was reported that muscle stiffness diminished, gross motor function improved and tone measured with MAS decreased after BoNT/A injection to gastrocnemius muscle combined with physiotherapy including electro stimulation, stretching and strengthening exercises applied twice a day for 4 weeks [70]. In another study conducted on children with spastic diparetic CP with the same design, it was reported that intrinsic stiffness of muscles decreased at the end of 4 weeks [77]. Some authors discussed that spastic muscle relaxation facilitates extremity growth and decreases fixed contracture development [57, 77, 78].

In animal experiments, it was shown that muscle and tendon growth and function was close to normal following BoNT/A injection; however, it caused reduction in bone mineral density [79]. It was reported that in some animals, BoNT/A injections made to nonspastic muscles prevented normal growth of muscle and caused progressive and persistent atrophy of muscle. In another study, it was reported that atrophy caused by BoNT/A injection was not reversed by exercise training [80, 81]. There are studies reporting that injections can cause decrease in muscle strength in children with CP; nevertheless, it was reported that there was 4–5% decrease in muscle volume by injections made to gastrocnemius muscle in 15 children with CP, and this was not as dramatic as in animal experiments [73, 82]. It was reported that

http://dx.doi.org/10.5772/66693

BoNT/A injections change muscle tone in the active, nonfibrotic and noncontractured sections of muscle and allowed stretching of muscle by decreasing tone, and this in turn was a stimulus for muscle growth. It was indicated that BoNT/A injection decreases agonist activity, supports antagonistic activity and must be combined with therapy to improve function, activity, participation and motor development in children with CP [34].

12. Age range

Spasticity develops in the first few years in children with CP. BoNT/A injections are suggested during 2–6 years of age while walking patterns and motor functions are prone to development [28]. According to a study conducted on 189 children with spastic CP in 2011, it was reported that the increase in dorsiflexion angle following BoNT/A injections made to triceps sure depended on the injected dosage and patient's age. It was reported that the obtained effect was as good as the children was younger [83]. There are limited reports about the usage of BoNT/A injections before 2 years of age. Usage in cases of 1 year 10 months of age was reported as the earliest [35]. BoNT/A was applied in children with CP younger than 2 years of age in very few studies, and in these studies, the effectiveness of the application was not analyzed separately for these children. Information is needed about the potential benefits or reliability in this age group [79].

13. Side effects

There are numerous studies scrutinizing the therapeutic benefits of BoNT/A injections in children with CP; however, there are limited publications about their safety. There were side effects observed depending on the application in 1–2% of children who were applied BoNT/A injections. Some authors consider neutralizing antibodies as responsible for side effects that develop after toxin injection. Formation of these substances increases BoNT/A amount that needs to be applied in the next injection. However, a single injection is not sufficient for many children and the injections need to be repeated in intervals of approximately 6 month intervals. In a research, it was reported that 58% of 4000 injections made during 15 years were first injections, 42% were second and the following [35].

In various researches, side effects of BoNT/A injections were reported as flu-like symptoms, nausea, diplopia, dysphagia, aspiration, respiratory tract infection, bronchitis, pharyngitis, pneumonia, asthma, generalized weakness, muscle weakness, urinary incontinence, falls, seizures, fever and unspecified pain [27, 84]. The start of systemic reactions can vary between the moment right after injection to a few weeks. There are studies reporting that urinary incontinence disappeared within 1–6 weeks. A relationship was found between BoNT/A dosage and hospitalization due to respiratory or urinary problems. It was reported that urinary and pulmonary problems that developed could be caused by systemic spread [35].

General anesthesia can increase side effects because anesthesia is a major risk factor for aspiration and infection. It could be difficult to distinguish whether the side effects occurred from BoNT/A or general anesthesia in the applications made under general anesthesia [35, 85].

It was reported that severity of the side effects related with the toxin was low; however, the number of side effects in children with CP were higher in comparison to other users. There are only a few studies reporting mortality following BoNT/A injections [86]. In literature, there are many studies about the positive effects of injection; however, there is inadequate information about optimal dosage, injection schemes and safety concerns [54].

Although injections generally have a good safety profile in short term, it is not suggested to use high doses in patients who have epilepsy or immune problems. It was reported that the children who were at level IV–V in GMFCS and had laryngeal and pharyngeal dysfunction were under more risk in terms of side effects [35, 85]. Further studies are needed to determine the relationship between especially mortality and epilepsy and BoNT/A injections [84].

The start of systemic reactions can vary between the moment right after injection to a few weeks. General anesthesia can increase side effects because anesthesia is the major risk factor for aspiration and infection. It could be difficult to distinguish whether the side effect stem from BoNT/A or general anesthesia in the applications made under general anesthesia [85].

In this section, it is understood that BoNT/A is a safe tool to decrease muscle tone in children with spastic CP and are effective in improving gross motor functions of children when combined with PT, OT, serial casting and orthesis. The injections have relatively few side effects, caring about patient selection and the dose to be applied should minimize side effects of the application. Further studies are needed to clarify what type of changes the injections cause in the architecture of spastic muscle in children with CP. Children with CP must be treated in a multidisciplinary setting where many specialists work together by combining many treatment approaches.

Author details

Ayse Numanoğlu Akbas

Address all correspondence to: aysenumanoglu@gmail.com

Department of Physical Therapy and Rehabilitation, Abant İzzet Baysal University, Bolu, Turkey

References

[1] Koman, L.A., et al., *Management of cerebral palsy with botulinum-A toxin: preliminary investigation.* Journal of Pediatric Orthopaedics, 1993. **13**(4): pp. 489–495.

[2] Cans, C., *Surveillance of cerebral palsy in Europe: a collaboration of cerebral palsy surveys and registers.* Developmental Medicine & Child Neurology, 2000. **42**(12): pp. 816–824.

[3] Rosenbaum, P., et al., *A report: the definition and classification of cerebral palsy April 2006.* Dev Med Child Neurol Suppl, 2007. **109**(suppl 109): pp. 8–14.

[4] Reddihough, D.S. and K.J. Collins, *The epidemiology and causes of cerebral palsy*. Australian Journal of physiotherapy, 2003. **49**(1): pp. 7–12.

[5] Bax, M.C., *Terminology and classification of cerebral palsy*. Developmental Medicine & Child Neurology, 1964. **6**(3): pp. 295–297.

[6] Ahlin, K., et al., *Cerebral palsy and perinatal infection in children born at term*. Obstetrics & Gynecology, 2013. **122**(1): pp. 41–49.

[7] Krigger, K.W., *Cerebral palsy: an overview*. Am Fam Physician, 2006. **73**(1): pp. 91–100.

[8] Europe, S.o.C.P.i. *CP and CP subtypes*. [cited 2015 29.06.2015]; Available from: http://www.scpenetwork.eu/en/my-scpe/rtm/cp-and-cp-subtypes/.

[9] Shumway-Cook, A. and M.H. Woollacott, *Motor control: theory and practical applications*. 1995: Lippincott Williams & Wilkins.

[10] Miller, F., *Physical therapy of cerebral palsy*. 2007.

[11] Elovic, E.P., L.K. Simone, and R. Zafonte, *Outcome assessment for spasticity management in the patient with traumatic brain injury: the state of the art*. The Journal of Head Trauma Rehabilitation, 2004. **19**(2): pp. 155–177.

[12] Sheean, G., *The pathophysiology of spasticity*. European Journal of Neurology, 2002. **9**(s1): pp. 3–9.

[13] Priori, A., F. Cogiamanian, and S. Mrakic-Sposta, *Pathophysiology of spasticity*. Neurological Sciences, 2006. **27**(4): pp. s307–s309.

[14] Quinby, J.M. and A. Abraham, *Musculoskeletal problems in cerebral palsy*. Current Paediatrics, 2005. **15**(1): pp. 9–14.

[15] Chaturvedi, S.K., et al., *Comparative assessment of therapeutic response to physiotherapy with or without botulinum toxin injection using diffusion tensor tractography and clinical scores in term diplegic cerebral palsy children*. Brain and Development, 2013. **35**(7): pp. 647–653.

[16] Thomas, R.E., et al., *GRIN: "GRoup versus INdividual physiotherapy following lower limb intra-muscular Botulinum Toxin-A injections for ambulant children with cerebral palsy: an assessor-masked randomised comparison trial": study protocol*. BMC Pediatrics, 2014. **14**(1): p. 1.

[17] Jianjun, L., et al., *Botulinum toxin-A with and without rehabilitation for the treatment of spastic cerebral palsy*. Journal of International Medical Research, 2013. **41**(3): pp. 636–641.

[18] Panteliadis, C.P., *Cerebral palsy*. 2004: Dustri-Verlag.

[19] Desloovere, K., et al., *The effect of different physiotherapy interventions in post-BTX-A treatment of children with cerebral palsy*. European Journal of Paediatric Neurology, 2012. **16**(1): pp. 20–28.

[20] Placzek, R., D. Siebold, and J.F. Funk, *Development of treatment concepts for the use of botulinum toxin a in children with cerebral palsy*. Toxins, 2010. **2**(9): pp. 2258–2271.

[21] Speth, L., et al., *Botulinum toxin A and upper limb functional skills in hemiparetic cerebral palsy: a randomized trial in children receiving intensive therapy.* Developmental Medicine & Child Neurology, 2005. **47**(7): pp. 468–473.

[22] Park, E.S., et al., *The effect of botulinum toxin type A injection into the gastrocnemius muscle on sit-to-stand transfer in children with spastic diplegic cerebral palsy.* Clinical Rehabilitation, 2006. **20**(8): pp. 668–674.

[23] Love, S., et al., *The effect of botulinum toxin type A on the functional ability of the child with spastic hemiplegia a randomized controlled trial.* European Journal of Neurology, 2001. **8**(s5): pp. 50–58.

[24] Russo, R.N., et al., *Upper-limb botulinum toxin A injection and occupational therapy in children with hemiplegic cerebral palsy identified from a population register: a single-blind, randomized, controlled trial.* Pediatrics, 2007. **119**(5): pp. e1149–e1158.

[25] Tedroff, K., et al., *Botulinumtoxin A treatment in toddlers with cerebral palsy.* Acta Paediatrica, 2010. **99**(8): pp. 1156–1162.

[26] O'Neil, M.E., M.A. Fragala, and H.M. Dumas, *Physical therapy intervention for children with cerebral palsy who receive botulinum toxin a injections.* Pediatric Physical Therapy, 2003. **15**(4): pp. 204–215.

[27] Love, S., et al., *Botulinum toxin assessment, intervention and after-care for lower limb spasticity in children with cerebral palsy: international consensus statement.* European Journal of Neurology, 2010. **17**(s2): pp. 9–37.

[28] Molenaers, G., et al., *The use of botulinum toxin A in children with cerebral palsy, with a focus on the lower limb.* Journal of Children's Orthopaedics, 2010. **4**(3): pp. 183–195.

[29] English, C.K., et al., *Circuit class therapy versus individual physiotherapy sessions during inpatient stroke rehabilitation: a controlled trial.* Archives of Physical Medicine and Rehabilitation, 2007. **88**(8): pp. 955–963.

[30] Galvin, J., et al., *Does intervention using virtual reality improve upper limb function in children with neurological impairment: a systematic review of the evidence.* Brain Injury, 2011. **25**(5): pp. 435–442.

[31] Novak, I., A. Cusick, and N. Lannin, *Occupational therapy home programs for cerebral palsy: double-blind, randomized, controlled trial.* Pediatrics, 2009. **124**(4): pp. e606–e614.

[32] Palisano, R., et al., *Development and reliability of a system to classify gross motor function in children with cerebral palsy.* Developmental Medicine & Child Neurology, 1997. **39**(4): pp. 214–223.

[33] García Salazar, L.F., et al., *Intrinsic properties and functional changes in spastic muscle after application of BTX-A in children with cerebral palsy: systematic review.* Developmental Neurorehabilitation, 2015. **18**(1): pp. 1–14.

[34] Heinen, F., et al., *The updated European Consensus 2009 on the use of Botulinum toxin for children with cerebral palsy.* European Journal of Paediatric Neurology, 2010. **14**(1): pp. 45–66.

[35] Naidu, K., et al., *Systemic adverse events following botulinum toxin A therapy in children with cerebral palsy.* Developmental Medicine & Child Neurology, 2010. **52**(2): pp. 139–144.

[36] Thorley, M., et al., *Evaluation of the effects of botulinum toxin A injections when used to improve ease of care and comfort in children with cerebral palsy whom are non-ambulant: a double blind randomized controlled trial.* BMC Pediatrics, 2012. **12**(1): p. 120.

[37] Tüzün, E.H., D.K. Guven, and L. Eker, *Pain prevalence and its impact on the quality of life in a sample of Turkish children with cerebral palsy.* Disability and Rehabilitation, 2010. **32**(9): pp. 723–728.

[38] Scholtes, V.A., et al., *The combined effect of lower-limb multilevel botulinum toxin type A and comprehensive rehabilitation on mobility in children with cerebral palsy: a randomized clinical trial.* Archives of Physical Medicine and Rehabilitation, 2006. **87**(12): pp. 1551–1558.

[39] Desloovere, K., et al., *Botulinum toxin type A treatment in children with cerebral palsy: evaluation of treatment success or failure by means of goal attainment scaling.* European Journal of Paediatric Neurology, 2012. **16**(3): pp. 229–236.

[40] Mikov, A., et al., *Use of botulinum toxin type A in children with spastic cerebral palsy.* HealthMED, 2011. **5**: pp. 922–928.

[41] Lee, S.J., et al., *The effect and complication of botulinum toxin type A injection with serial casting for the treatment of spastic equinus foot.* Annals of Rehabilitation Medicine, 2011. **35**(3): pp. 344–353.

[42] Van der Houwen, L., et al., *Botulinum toxin A injections do not improve surface EMG patterns during gait in children with cerebral palsy—A randomized controlled study.* Gait & Posture, 2011. **33**(2): pp. 147–151.

[43] Unlu, E., et al., *Multilevel botulinum toxin type a as a treatment for spasticity in children with cerebral palsy: a retrospective study.* Clinics, 2010. **65**(6): pp. 613–619.

[44] Lukban, M.B., R.L. Rosales, and D. Dressler, *Effectiveness of botulinum toxin A for upper and lower limb spasticity in children with cerebral palsy: a summary of evidence.* Journal of Neural Transmission, 2009. **116**(3): pp. 319–331.

[45] Ryll, U., et al., *Effects of leg muscle botulinum toxin A injections on walking in children with spasticity-related cerebral palsy: a systematic review.* Developmental Medicine & Child Neurology, 2011. **53**(3): pp. 210–216.

[46] Ferrari, A., et al., *A randomized trial of upper limb botulimun toxin versus placebo injection, combined with physiotherapy, in children with hemiplegia.* Research in Developmental Disabilities, 2014. **35**(10): pp. 2505–2513.

[47] Sakzewski, L., J. Ziviani, and R.N. Boyd, *Efficacy of upper limb therapies for unilateral cerebral palsy: a meta-analysis.* Pediatrics, 2013: p. peds. 2013–0675.

[48] Novak, I., et al., *A systematic review of interventions for children with cerebral palsy: state of the evidence.* Developmental Medicine & Child Neurology, 2013. **55**(10): pp. 885–910.

[49] Speth, L., et al., *Effects of botulinum toxin A and/or bimanual task-oriented therapy on upper extremity activities in unilateral Cerebral Palsy: a clinical trial.* BMC Neurology, 2015. **15**(1): p. 1.

[50] Hoare, B.J., et al., *Constraint-induced movement therapy in the treatment of the upper limb in children with hemiplegic cerebral palsy.* Cochrane Database of Systematic Reviews, 2007. **2**.

[51] Hoare, B., et al., *Botulinum toxin A as an adjunct to treatment in the management of the upper limb in children with spastic cerebral palsy (UPDATE)(Review).* Cochrane Database of Systematic Reviews, 2010. **1**: p. CD003469.

[52] Hoare, B., et al., *Intensive therapy following upper limb botulinum toxin A injection in young children with unilateral cerebral palsy: a randomized trial.* Developmental Medicine & Child Neurology, 2013. **55**(3): pp. 238–247.

[53] Lidman, G., et al., *Botulinum toxin A injections and occupational therapy in children with unilateral spastic cerebral palsy: a randomized controlled trial.* Developmental Medicine & Child Neurology, 2015. **57**(8): pp. 754–761.

[54] Friedman, B.-C. and R.D. Goldman, *Use of botulinum toxin A in management of children with cerebral palsy.* Canadian Family Physician, 2011. **57**(9): pp. 1006–1073.

[55] Alhusaini, A.A., et al., *No change in calf muscle passive stiffness after botulinum toxin injection in children with cerebral palsy.* Developmental Medicine & Child Neurology, 2011. **53**(6): pp. 553–558.

[56] Lodha, N., et al., *Force control and degree of motor impairments in chronic stroke.* Clinical Neurophysiology, 2010. **121**(11): pp. 1952–1961.

[57] Bohannon, R.W. and M.B. Smith, *Interrater reliability of a modified Ashworth scale of muscle spasticity.* Physical Therapy, 1987. **67**(2): pp. 206–207.

[58] Haugh, A., A. Pandyan, and G. Johnson, *A systematic review of the Tardieu Scale for the measurement of spasticity.* Disability and Rehabilitation, 2006. **28**(15): pp. 899–907.

[59] Bar-On, L., et al., *Is an instrumented spasticity assessment an improvement over clinical spasticity scales in assessing and predicting the response to integrated botulinum toxin type A treatment in children with cerebral palsy?* Archives of Physical Medicine and Rehabilitation, 2014. **95**(3): pp. 515–523.

[60] Scholtes, V.A., et al., *Clinical assessment of spasticity in children with cerebral palsy: a critical review of available instruments.* Developmental Medicine & Child Neurology, 2006. **48**(1): pp. 64–73.

[61] Flamand, V.H., H. Massé-Alarie, and C. Schneider, *Psychometric evidence of spasticity measurement tools in cerebral palsy children and adolescents: a systematic review.* Journal of Rehabilitation Medicine, 2013. **45**(1): pp. 14–23.

[62] Jethwa, A., et al., *Development of the Hypertonia Assessment Tool (HAT): a discriminative tool for hypertonia in children.* Developmental Medicine & Child Neurology, 2010. **52**(5): pp. e83–e87.

[63] Leonard, C.T., J.U. Stephens, and S.L. Stroppel, *Assessing the spastic condition of individuals with upper motoneuron involvement: validity of the myotonometer.* Archives of Physical Medicine and Rehabilitation, 2001. **82**(10): pp. 1416–1420.

[64] Syczewska, M., M.K. Lebiedowska, and A.D. Pandyan, *Quantifying repeatability of the Wartenberg pendulum test parameters in children with spasticity.* Journal of Neuroscience Methods, 2009. **178**(2): pp. 340–344.

[65] Boiteau, M., F. Malouin, and C.L. Richards, *Use of a hand-held dynamometer and a Kin-Com® dynamometer for evaluating spastic hypertonia in children: a reliability study.* Physical Therapy, 1995. **75**(9): pp. 796–802.

[66] van den Noort, J.C., V.A. Scholtes, and J. Harlaar, *Evaluation of clinical spasticity assessment in cerebral palsy using inertial sensors.* Gait & Posture, 2009. **30**(2): pp. 138–143.

[67] Schmartz, A.C., et al., *Measurement of muscle stiffness using robotic assisted gait orthosis in children with cerebral palsy: a proof of concept.* Disability and Rehabilitation: Assistive Technology, 2011. **6**(1): pp. 29–37.

[68] Kohan, A.H., et al., *Comparison of modified Ashworth scale and Hoffmann reflex in study of spasticity.* Acta Medica Iranica, 2010. **48**(3): pp. 154–157.

[69] Poon, D.M. and C.W. Hui-Chan, *Hyperactive stretch reflexes, co-contraction, and muscle weakness in children with cerebral palsy.* Developmental Medicine & Child Neurology, 2009. **51**(2): pp. 128–135.

[70] Kwon, D.R., G.Y. Park, and J.G. Kwon, *The change of intrinsic stiffness in gastrocnemius after intensive rehabilitation with botulinum toxin A injection in spastic diplegic cerebral palsy.* Annals of Rehabilitation Medicine, 2012. **36**(3): pp. 400–403.

[71] Ackman, J.D., et al., *Comparing botulinum toxin A with casting for treatment of dynamic equinus in children with cerebral palsy.* Developmental Medicine & Child Neurology, 2005. **47**(9): pp. 620–627.

[72] Ubhi, T., et al., *Randomised double blind placebo controlled trial of the effect of botulinum toxin on walking in cerebral palsy.* Archives of Disease in Childhood, 2000. **83**(6): pp. 481–487.

[73] Williams, S.A., et al., *Muscle volume alterations in spastic muscles immediately following botulinum toxin type-A treatment in children with cerebral palsy.* Developmental Medicine & Child Neurology, 2013. **55**(9): pp. 813–820.

[74] El-Etribi, M., et al., *The effect of botulinum toxin type-A injection on spasticity, range of motion and gait patterns in children with spastic diplegic cerebral palsy: an Egyptian study.* International Journal of Rehabilitation Research, 2004. **27**(4): pp. 275–281.

[75] Baird, M.W. and J. Vargus-Adams, *Outcome measures used in studies of botulinum toxin in childhood cerebral palsy: a systematic review.* Journal of Child Neurology, 2010. **25**(6): pp. 721–727.

[76] Sugden, D. and M. Wade, *Typical and atypical motor development.* Adapted Physical Activity Quarterly, 2013. **30**: pp. 387–388.

[77] Park, G.-Y. and D.R. Kwon, *Sonoelastographic evaluation of medial gastrocnemius muscles intrinsic stiffness after rehabilitation therapy with botulinum toxin a injection in spastic cerebral palsy.* Archives of Physical Medicine and Rehabilitation, 2012. **93**(11): pp. 2085–2089.

[78] Cosgrove, A. and H. Graham, *Botulinum toxin A prevents the development of contractures in the hereditary spastc mouse.* Developmental Medicine & Child Neurology, 1994. **36**(5): pp. 379–385.

[79] Bakheit, A.M., *The use of botulinum toxin for the treatment of muscle spasticity in the first 2 years of life.* International Journal of Rehabilitation Research, 2010. **33**(2): pp. 104–108.

[80] Velders, M., et al., *Effect of botulinum toxin A-induced paralysis and exercise training on mechanosensing and signalling gene expression in juvenile rat gastrocnemius muscle.* Experimental Physiology, 2008. **93**(12): pp. 1273–1283.

[81] Chen, C.-M., N.S. Stott, and H.K. Smith, *Effects of botulinum toxin A injection and exercise on the growth of juvenile rat gastrocnemius muscle.* Journal of Applied Physiology, 2002. **93**(4): pp. 1437–1447.

[82] Gough, M., C. Fairhurst, and A. Shortland, *Botulinum toxin and cerebral palsy: time for reflection?* Developmental Medicine & Child Neurology, 2005. **47**(10): pp. 709–712.

[83] Pascual-Pascual, S.I., I. Pascual-Castroviejo, and P.J.G. Ruiz, *Treating spastic equinus foot from cerebral palsy with botulinum toxin type A: what factors influence the results?: an analysis of 189 consecutive cases.* American Journal of Physical Medicine & Rehabilitation, 2011. **90**(7): pp. 554–563.

[84] Albavera-Hernández, C., J.M. Rodríguez, and A.J. Idrovo, *Safety of botulinum toxin type A among children with spasticity secondary to cerebral palsy: a systematic review of randomized clinical trials.* Clinical Rehabilitation, 2009.

[85] Howell, K., et al., *Botulinum neurotoxin A: an unusual systemic effect.* Journal of Paediatrics and Child Health, 2007. **43**(6): pp. 499–501.

[86] Graham, H.K., et al., *Does botulinum toxin A combined with bracing prevent hip displacement in children with cerebral palsy and "hips at risk"?* The Journal of Bone & Joint Surgery, 2008. **90**(1): pp. 23–33.

Section 4

Botulinum Toxin Therapy: Instrument - Guidance

Chapter 9

How Can We Clinically Apply Ultrasound-Guided BoNT-A Injection Technology for Muscle Spasticity in Stroke Patients?

Li Jiang and Zulin Dou

Additional information is available at the end of the chapter

http://dx.doi.org/10.5772/66697

Abstract

In this chapter, the primary focus is towards four topics related to the ultrasound (US)-guided injection: (1) the advantages of various guided injection techniques including US-guided injection, (2) a brief review of recently published studies on the US-guided botulinum toxin type A (BoNT-A) injection in stroke patients, (3) standardized operational procedures for the US-guided injection and (4) a description of the skills necessary to properly locate the probe and limb during the US-guided injection operation. Illustrations will be presented in the chapter to assist the readers in gaining a better understanding of the US-guided BoNT-A injection technique.

Keywords: botulinum toxin type A, spasticity, post-stroke, ultrasound

1. Introduction

In the post-stroke rehabilitation setting, botulinum toxin type A (BoNT-A) represents a first-line treatment for focal spasticity. Botulinum toxin type A is regarded as an effective treatment agent, and the efficacy and safety of BoNT-A injected in post-stroke patients with lower limb spasticity have been suggested in a few limited-scale randomized controlled trials [1, 2], as well as a meta-analysis study [3]. A successful and safe therapy using BoNT-A requires an anatomically accurate administration of BoNT-A into the muscles of the belly. One should be aware that BoNT-A may induce undue weakness to adjacent unaffected muscles. Knowing the location of the needle can help clinicians more accurately inject BoNT-A into the target muscle. To date, manual needle placement (MNP), electromyography (EMG), electrical stimulation (ES) and ultrasound (US) guidance have all been applied during BoNT-A injection [4].

Moreover, there are less frequently used localization techniques that exist to include fluoroscopy, computed tomography (CT) and endoscopic guidance. As a clinician, one should be knowledgeable of the characteristics regarding the localized injection technique and the disadvantages and advantage of each injection technique. Then, the clinician can determine the appropriate localization technique that is specifically designed for the patient under examination. The issues related to injection techniques will be discussed in the following chapter.

2. Comparisons of different guided injection techniques for BoNT-A

2.1. Manual needle placement

As presented above, there are four types of localization techniques that are traditionally used in clinical practice. Manual needle placement, also referred to as anatomical localization, is the simplest type of localization technique. This technique does not require the use of any equipment, unlike the other three above-mentioned localization techniques. When using MNP for injection, the clinician should be knowledgeable of the positions of the bones in the procedural area of the body and use palpation to identify the target muscles. To correctly inject patients, the physician should have a thorough understanding of the anatomical position of the target muscle as well as the surrounding muscles. Texts provide electromyographers with consistent electrode insertion sites for each muscle [5]. Following these same insertion sites of electrography, physicians can locate the target muscles. Sometimes, in order to verify the location better, the physician should use some manoeuvres and indirect signs emitted from passive palpation spastic muscles prior to injection.

There are several advantages of MNP localization. The most apparent advantage of this technique is that no equipment is required. A small-gauge needle is used to complete the injection instead of the larger-gauge needles that are required with EMG or ES injection. Moreover, the use of a smaller needle may decrease the level of discomfort. In addition, MNP localization is a relatively quick method that can be utilized to reduce the injection duration. Several disadvantages surface when MNP localization is used alone. The large, superficial muscles may be easily distinguishable with anatomic localization alone; however, other small, deeper muscles may not be as easily identified. Further, the spastic muscles can atrophy or twist, and these conditions can potentially alter the anatomical location of the muscle itself. In some cases, patients are unable to have a standard position that is appropriate for injection as demonstrated by the electrography tests. These conditions result in MNP localization as the suboptimal localization [6]. Henzel et al. [7] demonstrated this concept to determine whether US localization is equivalent to anatomical localization in order to identify BoNT-A injection targets. The investigators were able to locate the forearm spastic muscle using two separate localization techniques. The study results showed that significant differences were observed between MNP localization and US localization for several flexor muscles. This group believed that the landmark measurement was based on cadaveric studies and that it is difficult to place patients with spasticity in a standard supination and extension position. Furthermore, in the case of in-patients with spasticity, the typical three-dimensional structure of the forearm may be distorted due to severe muscle atrophy [8].

2.2. Electromyography-guided injection

The EMG-guided injection technique is familiar amongst many physicians who treat spasticity using BoNT-A. This injection technique has the ability to precisely identify spastic muscles and requires an EMG machine and a hollow insulated monopolar needle electrode [6]. To conduct this technique, the physician first ensures that the target muscles align with the anatomical localization and then administers the EMG-guided injection. Once the EMG needle electrode is inserted into spastic muscle, the physician should hear the involuntary motor unit action potentials (MUAPs), which may initially have a dull muffled sound, but will become sharper as the needle is advanced closer to the end plate. In order to make sure that the spastic muscle is correctly targeted, the physician may ask the patient to move that muscle, and the physician will then listen for increased signalling of MUAPs. In the event that the patient is unable to voluntarily contract the muscle using active motions, the physician may conduct a passive range of motion (PROM) to stretch the target muscle in the patient [9].

There are several advantages that are associated with the use of EMG-guided injection. An auditory EMG device is inexpensive and provides a mechanism for more precisely localizing the spastic target muscles. In addition, the EMG-guided injection is helpful for the delivery of the BoNT-A near the motor endplate of the spastic muscle or in the location of a high concentration of active MUAPs [10, 11]. There are a few disadvantages associated with EMG-guided technique. At first, this technique does not guarantee that the monopolar needle is inserted in the target muscle. Voluntary activation and PROM are used to decrease this risk; however, for deeper or overlapping muscles, there would be a greater probability for misplacement of the needle. In some instances, the physician may inject into a spastic muscle that may not be the target muscle. To circumvent these issues, the clinician may increase the frequency and intensity of the muscle stimulus to identify spastic muscle, which may extend the time duration of the procedure and intensify the level of pain as compared with anatomic guidance. Other disadvantages of the EMG-guided injection technique are the costs of the insulated EMG needle and the costs of the EMG machine compare with anatomic guidance [6].

2.3. Electrical stimulation-guided injection

The electrical stimulation-guided injection is a popular technique for muscle localization. In this method, like EMG-guided injection, a hollow insulated monopolar needle is connected to a portable ES machine, and the target muscle is located by anatomical landmarks. Once the needle electrode is located in the target muscle, electric current is delivered to the muscle through the needle electrode. Normally, a 5-mA stimulus at 1-Hz intervals is applied to contract the muscle. Once the level of muscle contraction is identified as appropriate, the clinician may attempt to maintain a robust contraction while slowly decreasing the intensity of the muscle stimulation or incrementally modify the needle electrode, as needed. If the clinician is able to maintain the muscle contraction using a low-intensity stimulus, such as a 1 mA, the clinician can be relatively certain that the tip of the needle is proximal to the motor endplate [6].

One advantage of the ES-guided injection technique is the accuracy of the targeted muscle localization. The visual feedback from the spastic muscle contraction ensures that the needle is properly inserted in the target muscle, especially in the event that muscle contraction occurs under a low-intensity stimulus. The disadvantage of using the ES-guided technique to locate the target muscle is that this technique may result in increased time consumption and may require additional training compared to the other techniques mentioned herein. Moreover, this technique may cause the patient to experience a higher level of discomfort than the other techniques. In addition to the disadvantages of the ES-guided technique, for patients with severe spasticity and limited range of motion, it may be difficult to assess individual muscle contraction. Lastly, the costs of both the needle electrode and the ES device must be considered in clinical practice when conducting this method.

2.4. Ultrasound-guided injection

Ultrasonography is well established as a reliable and reproducible imaging method that is used to identify the anatomy of the muscle [12]. Ultrasound machines consist of several components: the transducer, the computer processor unit and the monitor. Transducers are available in high and low frequencies, while the higher-frequency transducers are used for more superficial structures at a high resolution and the lower-frequency transducers can be used to assess deeper structures. The clinician who is experienced with the use of US-guided injection is able to recognize the cross-sectional anatomy that is displayed on the monitor and is able to visualize the needle tip once it is injected into the target muscle.

There are many advantages of the US-guided injection with BoNT-A. This technique allows real-time visualization of the needle into structures including the target muscles and adjunct tissues. This method not only permits the clinician to more precisely identify the target muscles but also permits the avoidance of needle penetration in some other bodily structures, to include the blood vessels and nerves. Other potential benefits of this technique is that US-guided technique procedure is relatively more efficient with respect to the time needed to conduct this technique, and the patients experience less pain compared with the ES-guided and EMG-guided injections. The lowered pain indication can be attributed to the use of a smaller gauge needle [7]. In addition, the use of US-guided injection may help to reduce side effects of the injected medicine, such as the dissemination of BoNT-A into nontargeted areas. Moreover, the clinician is able to visualize the volume of the injected BoNT-A solution in real time and administer the appropriate amount of solution into the targeted muscle. This feature permits the physician to relocate the needle tip to a different area within the same target muscle in order to complete the injection and minimize the spread of the BoNT-A solution into the adjacent off-target muscles.

Although the US-guided injection technique for BoNT-A is regarded as the most accurate method for locating the target muscles, shortcomings exist for this technique. At first, operation of the US transducer and the syringe simultaneously may require the presence of an assistant. This is particularly necessary for the clinicians who are novel to this technique. It is advisable that clinicians who are interested in using the US guidance to localize the target muscle should seek the appropriate training in great sufficiency prior to administering this technique.

Which type of guided injection technique is most appropriate to eliminate toxins? Other investigators have reviewed and compared these guided injection techniques in details as reported in recent publications [4, 6, 13]. First, we believe that the clinicians who will perform

http://dx.doi.org/10.5772/66697

the BoNT-A injections for spasticity management should be knowledgeable of the advantages and disadvantages of each of the injection techniques as previously discussed. Second, the clinicians should undergo combined training experiences in order to adequately explain each technique in sufficient detail to the patient and ensure that the appropriate technique aligns with the needs of the patient. Finally, one should consider additional factors, such as equipment cost, spastic muscles location when considering the most appropriate guided injection technique. Although it seems that each of these localization techniques is superior to the use of anatomical localization alone, we believe that the anatomical localization should be the established standard when considering the use of an instrument-guided injection technique. Further, more studies are needed to determine which combination of localization techniques can produce the best clinical outcomes.

3. A review of the studies that administered US-guided BoNT-A injection into the upper and lower limb muscles of stroke patients

The use of US is a well-established reliable and reproducible imaging method for defining muscle anatomy. An ultrasound system with a 7.5-MHz linear transducer can provide sufficient resolution for both superficial and deep-seated muscles [14]. As an alternative to the electrophysiological techniques, US offers a visually controlled method of injection of BoNT-A [15, 16]. Schiano et al. were the first to report on the US-guided BoNT-A injection for the treatment of achalasia [17]. Since that time, the advantages of the US-guided BoNT-A injection have been recognized, and the use of this technique is becoming more widespread in the present years. In the previous years, Berweck and colleagues utilized US-guided injections for spastic muscles in children. From the years 2000 to 2003, these investigators administered over 6000 injections into 70 different muscles in a total of 350 children. Berweck et al. recommended the use of US to conduct anatomically precise injection of BoNT-A due to the advantageous features of sonography, which is easy, quick, painless and available in most hospitals [15, 16]. Until now, the use of US was mostly popular amongst pediatrics, and it seemed that the use of US was the obvious choice for spastic muscle identification and injection control [4].

Several studies suggested that the various guided BoNT-A injection techniques such as ES guided, EMG guided and US guided showed a greater spasticity reduction in conjunction with improved clinical outcomes when compared with MNP localization. In a clinical study conducted by Yang et al. [18], MNP into the gastrocnemius muscle (GCM) for BoNT-A injection in children with spastic cerebral palsy (CP) was investigated to analyze its accuracy and effectiveness. The accuracy of MNP by one researcher using anatomic landmarks alone was assessed by another researcher who used US visualization prior to BoNT-A injection. These researchers found that the MNP was accurately placed into the GCM in 78.7% of cases, with the greatest accuracy being with the needle insertion into the medial GCM (92.6%) and the lowest accuracy was observed in the lateral GCM (64.7%). These investigators reported that the lateral portion of the GCM was thinner than the medial GCM, and this resulted in a greater rate of misplaced needle. Injection of the BoNT-A into GCMs using an anatomical landmark was an acceptable approach for injection into the medial GCM; however, this approach was not effective when administered in the lateral GCM. Py et al. [19] evaluated the effectiveness of injecting BoNT-A into the lower limbs of children with CP using the needle placement technique (MNP or US guided). Thirty of the children received US-guided injections, and the remainder received injections using anatomical localization. These investigators evaluated the gait and the spasticity (Tardieu scale), a functional evaluation (the Gross Motor Function Measure) 4 weeks after the injection. Clinical effectiveness was noted in the children receiving US-guided injections compared with MNP alone, and the "functional effectiveness" was also improved in the children with the use of US. The results of the aforementioned studies support the concept that the US-guided injection is more effective than the MNP localization technique administered in the spastic muscles of patients with CP. In contrast to the study conducted by Py et al., Kwon et al. [20] evaluated the clinical outcomes in 32 children with CP following BoNT-A injections into the GCMs. These investigators compared the efficacy of ES guided and US guided for BoNT-A injections into the GCMs in the children. These researchers found no significant differences between the groups according to the scores on the modified Ashworth Scale scores (MAS) and the Modified Tardieu Scale (MTS) assessments; however, the subscales of the Physician's Rating Scale significantly improved in children who received BoNT-A injections when guided by US. Although similar results showed that spasticity levels between the US-guided injection and ES-guided injection were decreased, the investigators concluded that the visual feedback provided by the US-guided injection may improve the accuracy of the administration of BoNT-A into the GCMs in the children.

To date, a few studies have compared the precision of the MNP and US localization in efforts to identify the forearm flexor muscles that will undergo BoNT-A injections in subjects with arm spasticity. In an observational study of 18 adult patients with upper extremity spasticity, Henzel et al. [7] explored the accuracy of the MNP to locally administer the investigational agent in the forearm flexor muscles. After the measurements of the surface, marks were obtained, and US was used to determine the optimal injection site, which is described as the portion of the target muscle with the largest cross-sectional area. There was a statistically significant difference between the proposed injection sites as per the methods of MNP and the actual optimal injections sites as determined via the US-guided injections for the flexor pollicis longus, pronator teres and flexor digitorum superficialis (FDS) to digit 3, with trends towards significance in the flexor carpi radialis and FDS to digits 2 and 4. Based on these findings, the investigators recommend that the US-guided technique should be considered for muscle localization in patients with upper extremity spasticity. Picelli et al. [21] completed a single-blinded, randomized controlled study comparing the outcomes of 60 chronic stroke patients with clenched fist or flexed wrist who underwent BoNT-A injections with MNP or ES-guided or US-guided injections. Each subject underwent pre-injection and postinjection evaluations that included MAS, Tardieu angle and PROM. These investigators found enhanced improvement in all of the measurements when comparing the ES group with the MNP group. Likewise, the subjects in the US-guided BoNT-A injection group demonstrated greater improvement in all of the measurements when compared with the MNP group. There was no difference noted in the clinical outcomes when comparing patients who received injections when guided by ES versus the injections that were guided by US. These authors concluded that the use of ES- and US-guided BoNT-A injections decreases spasticity and results in vast improvements in the range of motion when compared to MNP techniques alone.

Santamato et al. [22] compared the reduction of spasticity and the related finger position at rest improvement in post-stroke patients treated with BoNT-A in the wrist and finger flexor limb muscles using US-guided injection and MNP localization. In the randomized clinical trial, two groups of 15 stroke patients were treated with BoNT-A injections in the wrist and finger flexor muscles of the affected upper limb using US-guided injections or MNP localization. The MAS and the finger position at rest were measured before and 4 weeks after administration of the injections. The results showed the MAS and finger position at rest significantly improved in both of the treatment groups, although these clinical outcomes were more effective in patients who received the US-guided BoNT-A injection compared to patients injected with BoNT-A using MNP localization. The investigators concluded that the US-guided BoNT-A injections were capable of improving the clinical outcome more effectively than MNP in post-stroke patients with spasticity.

In a study conducted by our team [23], we injected BoNT-A while being guided by US in patients with post-stroke wrist and finger flexor muscle spasticity and assessed the clinical outcomes following the injection and rehabilitation intervention. The results showed significant decreases in the MAS scores of both the finger flexor muscle and wrist flexor muscle at all time points after BoNT-A injections in comparison with the baseline scores. Compared with the baseline, the PROM of the wrist and finger extensions and the FMA scores of the wrist and hand significantly increased ($p < 0.001$) at 2, 4 and 12 weeks after the injections. We concluded that the US-guided injection of BoNT-A combined with rehabilitation exercise decreased the spasticity of the wrist and finger flexor muscles and improved the motor function in stroke patients up to 12 weeks following the BoNT-A injection.

Based on these aforementioned studies, all of the researchers have suggested that the US-guided injection technique is more effective in improving the accuracy of toxin placement in patients with limb spasticity. Most importantly, the US-guided injection is visually controlled. In viewing the entire process, the operator gains a better understanding of the anatomy of the individual under observation. This enables a more effective and safer technique selection and assists in the reduction of side effects due to the unintentional spread of medicine. Despite the fact that US cannot measure the muscular hyperactivity and detect motor endplate regions, the ultrasound images can provide information about muscle size and fibrosis, which are all factors that can be important in the decision-making process.

4. A description of the procedures for US-guided BoNT-A injection in clinical practices

In order to make US-guided injections feasible and effective in clinical practice, in accordance with the practice experience, the authors have developed a set of standardized operational procedures that include target muscle identification, the selected probe for upper and muscles images, the relationship between the limb and probe positioning, the proper needle types used for different muscles, the distance between the injecting needle and probe and needle tilting angle and the coordination between the operators and others involved in the injection process.

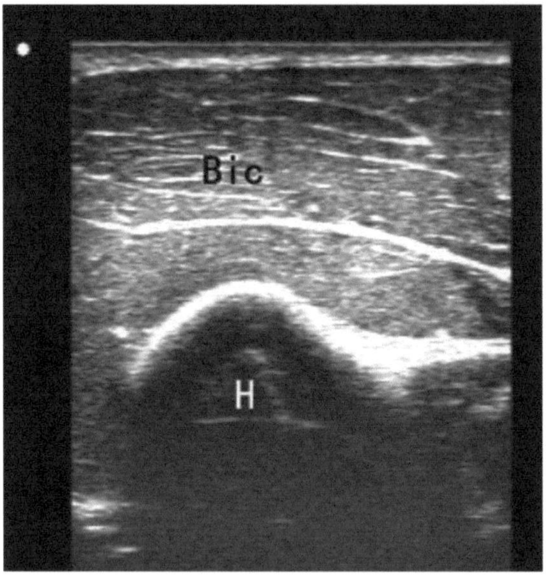

Figure 1. Sonographic image of the upper limb (Bic = bicep, H = humerus).

1. Probe selection

The 7.5-MHz linear transducer can provide sufficient resolution for superficial muscles but is also able to detect deep-seated muscles.

2. Probe viewing mode

The transverse viewing mode is arranged such that the medial part of the limb is seen on the right and the lateral part of the limb (the right side) is seen on the left side of the monitor screen.

3. Muscle imaging

The musculature appears poorly echogenic, while the perimysia and fascicular tissue between the muscle bellies are apparently echogenic. The two principles of muscle identification are (1) recognizing the characteristic pattern of the individual muscles. The transverse sonogram corresponds to the transverse anatomic sections. (2) Each muscle has a characteristic contour line. These muscles exhibit specific patterns and allow prompt (within a few seconds) identification of the individual muscles. An example for the upper or lower limb is shown in **Figures 1** and **2**.

4. Imaging of neighbouring structures

Visualization of the neighbouring structures, such as the bones and vessels, helps to accurately determine the injection site in target muscles. An example is shown in **Figure 3.**

5. Identification of target muscles

The suggested manner to identify target muscles includes the following: (1) The skin surface location for the target muscle was identified on the basis of the use of the specific anatomic landmarks from Delagi et al. [5] and was subsequently marked. (2) The transducer was located

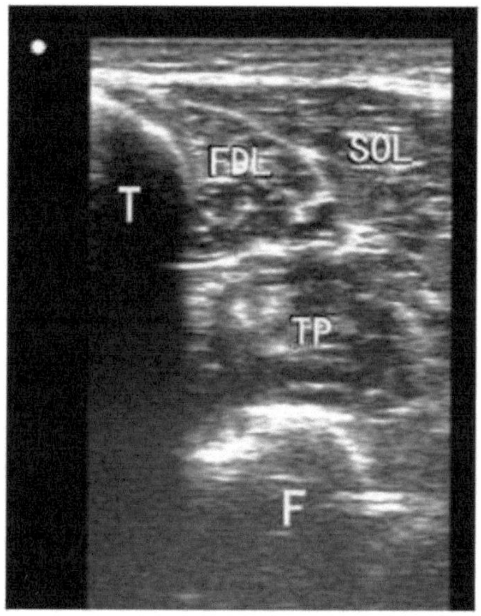

Figure 2. Sonographic image of the lower limb (SOL, soleus; FDL, flexor hallucis longus; TP, tibialis posterior; T, tibia; F, fibula).

at the marker and positioned perpendicularly to the skin surface to obtain a transverse view of the target muscle. (3) By adjusting the parameters such as view depth, focus and gain, a clear image of the target muscle and other muscles could be displayed (**Figures 4–6**).

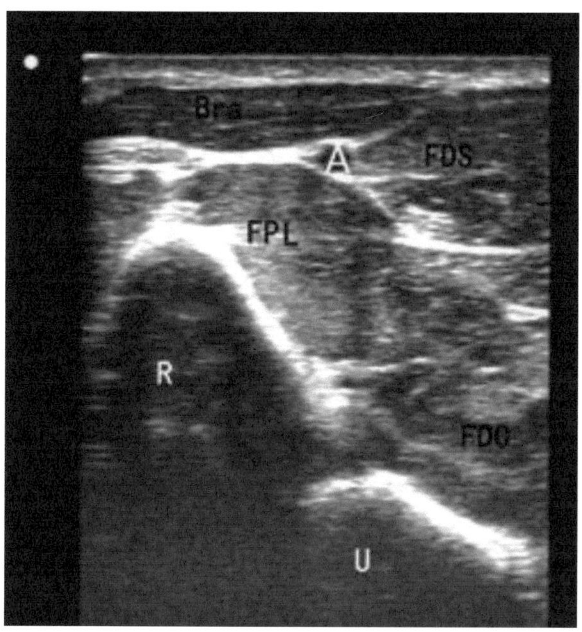

Figure 3. Sonographic image of the forearm, including the FDL and surrounding structures (Bra, brachioradialis; FPL, flexor pollicis longus; FDS, flexor digitorum superficialis; FDP, flexor digitorum profundus; A, artery; R, radius; U, ulna).

Note 1: Passive movements at small amplitudes are visible as concurrent oscillations of the intramuscular echo. Passive movement of the corresponding part of the body may help to visualize the dynamic contraction of the target muscle.

6. US-guided injection

To conduct the US-guided injection, (1) in the transverse (axial) view, the target muscle was scanned from the proximal to distal direction or vice versa until the largest cross-sectional area was identified. (2) The needle was inserted and was closely aligned to the longitudinal axis of the transducer (**Figure 7**). Slight movements of the needle along the transducer longitudinal axis are helpful to obtain a satisfactory image. (3) As the needle penetrates the skin, its path through the tissue to the target site for injection is continually monitored on the screen. (4) To confirm the surface injection site, in some cases, the second injection site of each target muscle was identified by distally moving the transducer approximately 1.5–2.0 cm. (5) Pre-injection sonographic images and the images during the injection are able to be stored for future references.

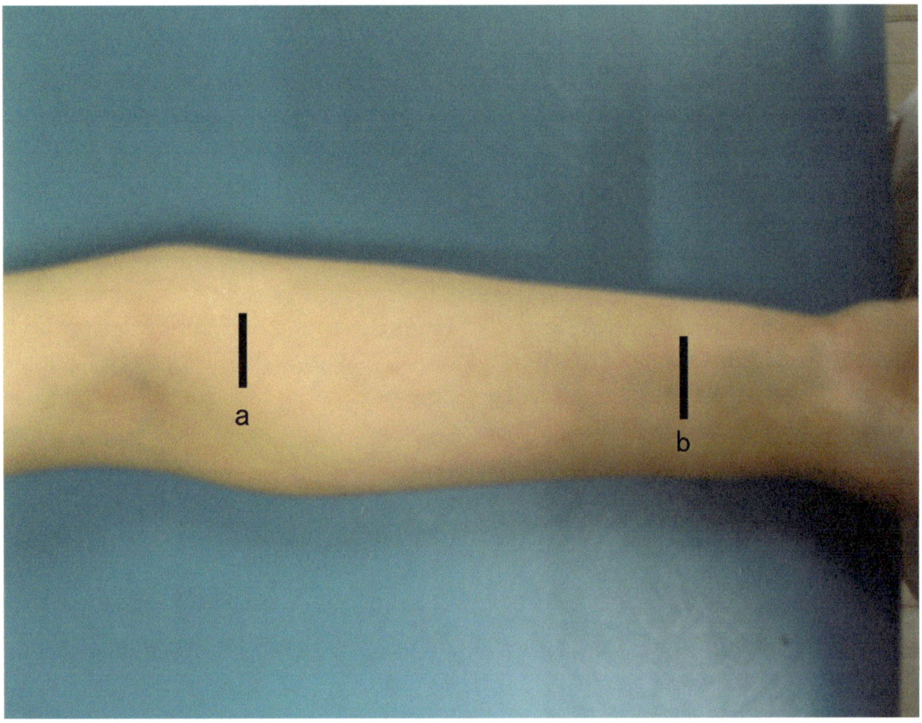

Figure 4. Probe location at different target muscles (a, pronator teres; b, pronator quadratus).

Upon injection, the solution spreads out in the muscle, usually as an echogenic cloud, sometimes with echo obliteration (**Figures 8** and **9**).

Note 2: Slight movements of the needle along its longitudinal axis can help to obtain a satisfactory image.

http://dx.doi.org/10.5772/66697

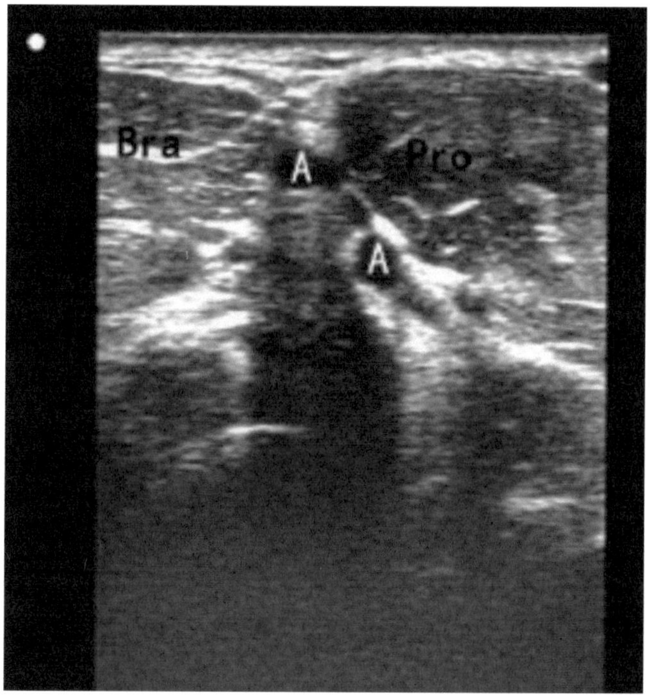

Figure 5. Sonographic image of the upper third of the anterior forearm (PT, pronator teres; Bra, brachioradialis; A, artery).

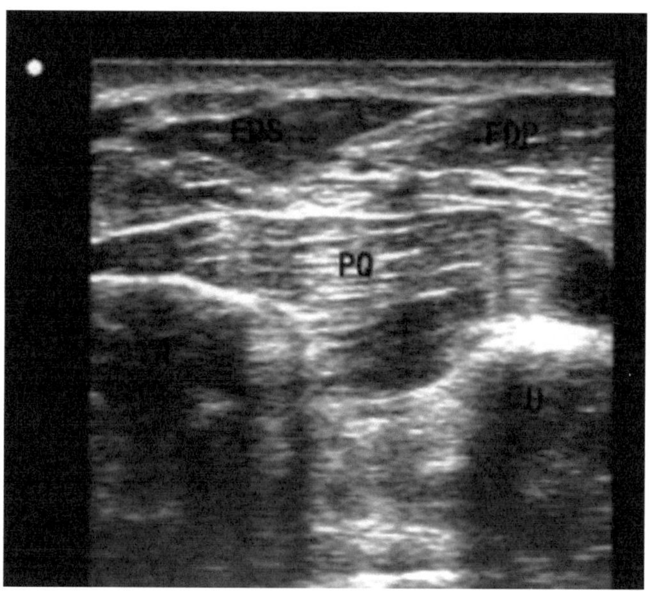

Figure 6. Sonographic image of the lower third portion of the anterior forearm (PQ, pronator quadratus; FDS, flexor digitorum superficialis; FDP, flexor digitorum profundus; R, radius; U, ulna).

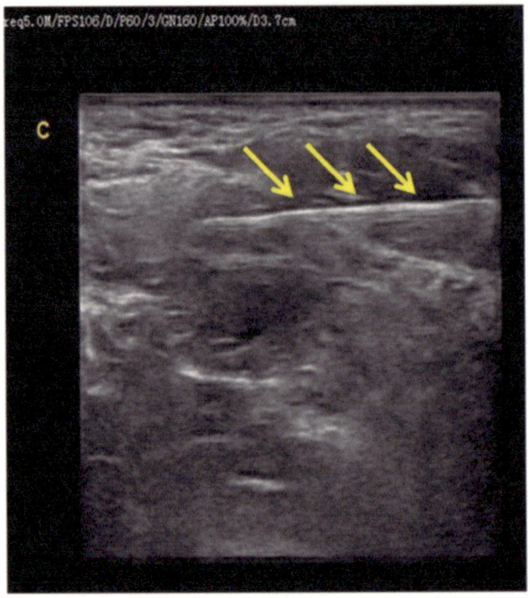

Figure 7. Sonographic image indicating the position of the inserted needle (arrow head points to the hyperecho line).

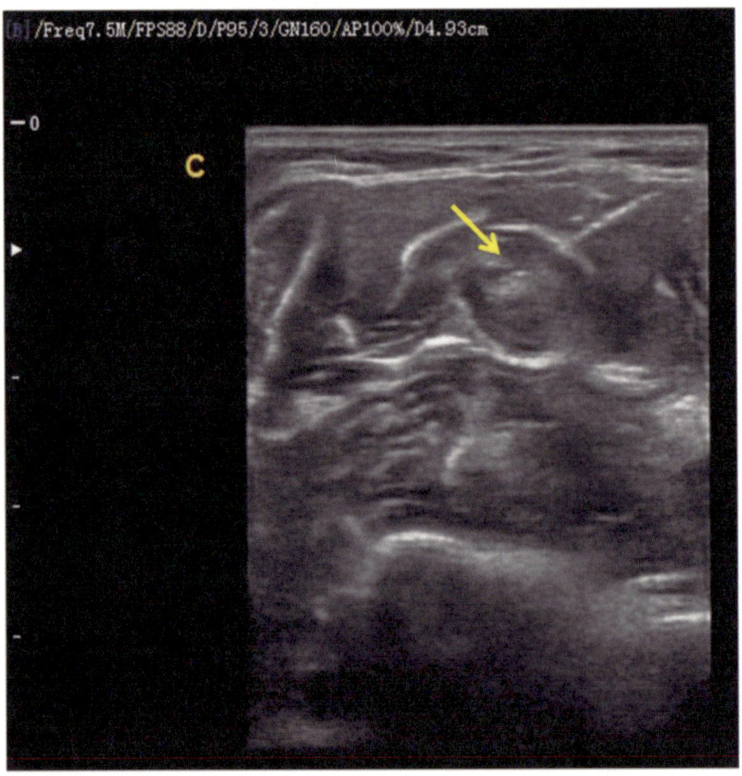

Figure 8. Needle in the target muscle before injection (arrow head points to the hyperecho point).

http://dx.doi.org/10.5772/66697

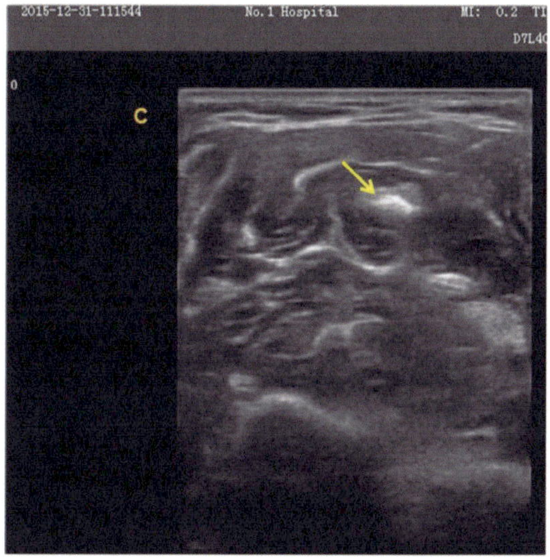

Figure 9. The solution disseminates into the target muscle (arrow head points to the hyperecho area).

5. A summary of the necessary skills to effectively administer the US-guided BoNT-A injection

1. Familiarity with the regional anatomy of the limb

It is well known that due to the size of the ultrasound probe, the pictures that are displayed on the screen of the ultrasound machine are specific only to the regional anatomy of the tissue under examination. Therefore, various probe locations result in different sonographic images. In order to achieve accurate injections, the clinician should undergo intense practice sessions in administering a variety of injections which will allow the clinician to become more familiar with the characteristics of the muscle and the surrounding structures as viewed through the sonographic machine. These practices are useful for precise injection into the target muscles and also ensure a safe and effective injection.

2. Basic operation of the ultrasound machine

The operators of the US machine should be competent in the use of this machine. A good understanding of the panel operation is helpful for adjusting the parameter settings in order to obtain the best image quality, which in turn would project the best injection site.

3. Spastic limb placement

In preparation of the injection, the injection site of the affected limb should be fully exposed. If patients with the higher spasticity levels are unable to position the limb appropriately, the clinician should ask for an assistant to help correctly position the limb.

4. The probe placement

The probe should be perpendicular to the plane of the proposed limb for injection. Proper probe placement is one of the basic requirements to obtain an excellent quality of ultrasound images. If the angle from the probe and body is too large or too small, the probe will receive sound reduction. Furthermore, the probe will produce unclear images of anatomical structure, and the accuracy of the injection will undergo severe alterations.

5. Relationship between the needle and probe (**Figures 10** and **11**)

In the in-plane position, the needle should be parallel to the probe. Next, the needle is inserted along the longitudinal axis of the probe. In this orientation, the needle is easy to visualize and the tip can be observed in its entirety during the injection.

In the out-of-plane position, the needle is inserted across the short axis of the probe at an angle to the skin. To properly conduct this technique, it is necessary to acquire the skills through repetitive practices and obtain a sufficient level of experience. The tip or shaft of the needle was seen as a hyper-echoic dot using the method.

The most common choice is the in-plane method in which the needle process can be observed throughout the muscle to ensure the safety and accuracy of the injection. In the out-of-plane position, the accuracy of injection may be affected due to the fact that only a portion of the needle is visible in the sonographic picture.

6. Ambidextrous coordination

As one hand holds the probe, the clinician should pay careful attention to the manner in which the probe is handled such that the probe is well positioned on the surface of the

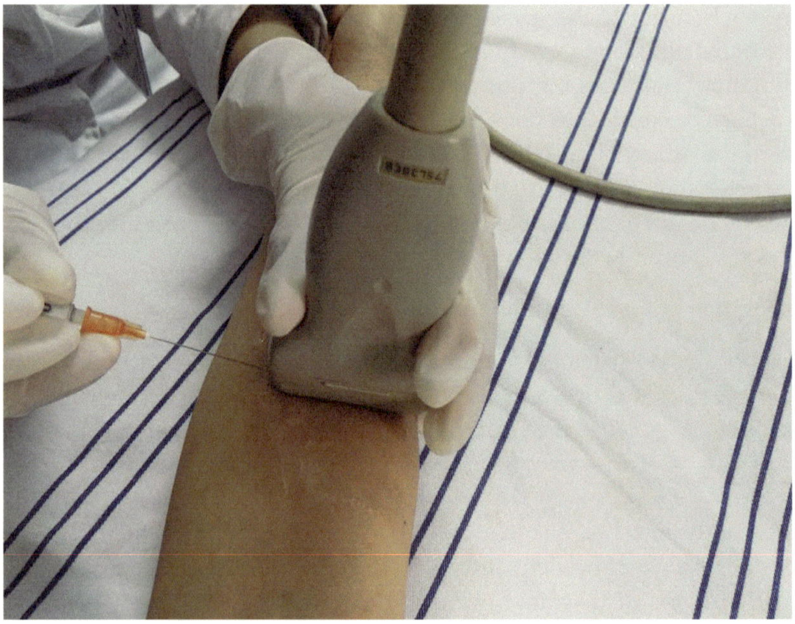

Figure 10. In plane (needle is parallel to probe).

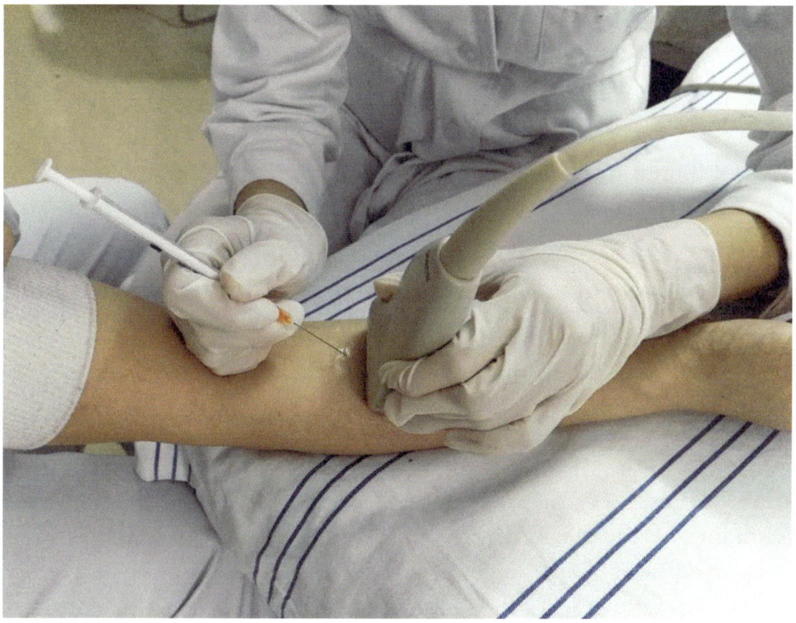

Figure 11. Out of plane (needle inserted across the short axis of probe).

skin. Using the other hand, the clinician is capable of the injection using the US-guided technique. For beginners, this ambidextrous coordination may seem challenging. With repetitive practices and increased exposure to this technique, the clinician will be able to master the skills.

7. Other skills

The operators involved with the injection procedure should practise sterile techniques.

Author details

Li Jiang* and Zulin Dou

*Address all correspondence to: 908455721@qq.com

Department of Rehabilitation Medicine, The Third Affiliated Hospital, Sun Yat-sen University, Guangzhou, China

References

[1] Farina, S., Migliorini, C., Gandolfi, M., Bertolasi, L., Casarotto, M., Manganotti, P., et al. Combined effects of botulinum toxin and casting treatments on lower limb spasticity after stroke. Funct Neurol. 2008, 23 (2): 87–91.

[2] Mancini, F., Sandrini, G., Moglia, A., Nappi, G., Pacchetti, C. A randomised, double-blind, dose-ranging study to evaluate efficacy and safety of three doses of botulinum toxin type A (Botox) for the treatment of spastic foot. Neurol Sci. 2005, 26 (1): 26–31.

[3] Rosales, R.L., Chua-Yap, A.S. Evidence-based systematic review on the efficacy and safety of botulinum toxin-A therapy in post-stroke spasticity. J Neural Transm. 2008, 115 (4): 617–623.doi: 10.1007/s00702-007-0869-3.

[4] Schroeder, A.S., Berweck, S., Lee, S.H., Heinen, F. Botulinum toxin treatment of children with cerebral palsy-a short review of different injection techniques. Neurotox Res. 2006, 9 (2–3): 189–196.

[5] Delagi, E.F., Perotto, A., Iazetti, J., Morrison, D. Anatomic Guide for the Electromyographer: The Limbs and Trunk. 4th ed. Springfield, IL: Charles C Thomas. Publisher, Ltd; 2005.

[6] Walker, H.W., Lee, M.Y., Bahroo, L.B., Hedera, P., Charles, D. Botulinum toxin injection techniques for the management of adult spasticity. PM R. 2014, 7 (4): 417–427. doi: 10.1016/j.pmrj.2014.09.021.

[7] Henzel, M.K., Munin M.C., Niyonkuru C., Skidmore E.R., Weber D.J., Zafonte R.D. Comparison of surface and ultrasound localization to identify forearm flexor muscles for botulinum toxin injections. PM R. 2010, 2 (7): 642–646. doi: 10.1016/j.pmrj.2010.05.002.

[8] Pillen, S., Arts, I.M., Zwarts, M.J. Muscle ultrasound in neuromuscular disorders. Muscle Nerve. 2008, 37 (6): 679–693. doi: 10.1002/mus.21015.

[9] O'Brien, C.F. Injection techniques for botulinum toxin using electromyography and electrical stimulation. Muscle Nerve Suppl. 1997, 6: S176–S180.

[10] Lapatki, B.G., van Dijk, J.P., van de Warrenburg, B.P., Zwarts, M.J. Botulinum toxin has an increased effect when targeted toward the muscle's endplate zone: a high-density surface EMG guided study. Clin Neurophysiol. 2011, 122 (8): 1611–1616. doi: 10.1016

[11] Gracies, J.M., Lugassy, M., Weisz, D.J., Vecchio, M., Flanagan, S., Simpson, D.M. Botulinum toxin dilution and endplate targeting in spasticity: a double-blind controlled study. Arch Phys Med Rehabil. 2009, 90 (1): 9–16.e2. doi: 10.1016.

[12] Fischer, A.Q., Carpenter, D.W., Hartlage, P.L., Carroll, J.E., Stephens, S. Muscle imaging in neuromuscular disease using computerized real-time sonography. Muscle Nerve. 1988, 11 (3): 270–275.

[13] Lim, E.C., Quek, A.M., Seet, R.C. Accurate targeting of botulinum toxin injections: how to and why. Parkinsonism Relat Disord. 2011, 17 (Suppl1): S34–S39. doi: 10.1016

[14] Willenborg, M.J., Shilt, J.S., Smith, B.P., Estrada, R.L., Castle, J.A., Koman, L.A. Technique for iliopsoas ultrasound-guided active electromyography-directed botulinum a toxin injection in cerebral palsy. J Pediatr Orthop. 2002, 22 (2): 165–168.

[15] Berweck, S., Feldkamp, A., Francke, A., Nehles, J., Schwerin, A., Heinen, F. Sonography-guided injection of botulinum toxin A in children with cerebral palsy. Neuropediatrics. 2002, 33 (4): 221–223.

[16] Berweck, S., Schroeder, A.S., Heinen, F. Sonography-guided injection of botulinum toxin in children with cerebral palsy. Lancet. 2004, 363 (9404): 249–250.

[17] Schiano, T.D., Fisher, R.S., Parkman, H.P., Cohen, S., Dabezies, M., Miller, L.S. Use of high-resolution endoscopic ultrasonography to assess esophageal wall damage after pneumatic dilation and botulinum toxin injection to treat achalasia. Gastrointest Endosc. 1996, 44 (2): 151–157.

[18] Yang, E.J., Rha, D.W., Yoo, J.K., Park, E.S. Accuracy of manual needle placement for gastrocnemius muscle in children with cerebral palsy checked against ultrasonography. Arch Phys Med Rehabil. 2009, 90 (5): 741–744. doi: 10.1016

[19] Py, A.G., Zein Addeen, G., Perrier, Y., Carlier, R.Y., Picard, A. Evaluation of the effectiveness of botulinum toxin injections in the lower limb muscles of children with cerebral palsy. Preliminary prospective study of the advantages of ultrasound guidance. Ann Phys Rehabil Med. 2009, 52 (3): 215–223.doi: 10.1016/j.rehab.2009.02.005.

[20] Kwon, J.Y., Hwang, J.H., Kim, J.S. Botulinum toxin a injection into calf muscles for treatment of spastic equinus in cerebral palsy: a controlled trial comparing sonography and electric stimulation-guided injection techniques: a preliminary report. Am J Phys Med Rehabil. 2010, 89 (4): 279–286. doi: 10.1097/PHM.0b013e3181ca24ac.

[21] Picelli, A., Lobba, D., Midiri, A., et al. Botulinum toxin injection into the forearm muscles for wrist and fingers spastic overactivity in adults with chronic stroke: a randomized controlled trial comparing three injection techniques. Clin Rehabil. 2014, 28 (3): 232–242. doi: 10.1177/0269215513497735.

[22] Santamato, A., Micello, M.F., Panza, F., Fortunato, F., Baricich, A., Cisari, C., Pilotto, A., Logroscino, G., Fiore, P., Ranieri, M. Can botulinum toxin type A injection technique influence the clinical outcome of patients with post-stroke upper limb spasticity? A randomized controlled trial comparing manual needle placement and ultrasound-guided injection techniques. J Neurol Sci. 2014, 15, 347 (1–2): 39–43. doi: 10.1016/j.jns.2014.09.016.

[23] Jiang, L., Dou, Z.L., Wang, Q., Wang, Q.Y., Dai, M., Wang, Z., Wei, X.M., Chen, Y.B. Evaluation of clinical outcomes of patients with post-stroke wrist and finger spasticity after ultrasonography-guided BTX-A injection and rehabilitation training. Front Hum Neurosci. 2015 Sep 2, 9: 485. doi: 10.3389/fnhum.2015.00485.

Chapter 10

How Useful are Localization Techniques in Botulinum Toxin Injections for Dystonia and Spasticity Indications?

Nikolina Ilkova Semerdjieva

Additional information is available at the end of the chapter

http://dx.doi.org/10.5772/64218

Abstract

There is irrefutable evidence for the effectiveness of botulinum toxin (BoNT) in the treatment of various disorders associated with excessive muscle contraction or autonomic dysfunction. One of the earliest indications as well as the most common BoNT treated movement disorder is dystonia, predominantly its focal forms, including blepharospasm, oromandibular, spasmodic, cervical and limb dystonia. Spastic disorders comprise another area where BoNT treatment has proved beneficial. Optimal therapeutic results, however, depend on several factors, including the BoNT serotype, dose, concentration, injected volume, frequency of application, as well as precise localization of the muscles producing the abnormal movement. The accuracy in targeting muscle localization is considered to be a key factor for determining the outcome of BoNT injections, even more important than dilution volume and dose. Various techniques to find the best injection site for the delivery of BoNT have been described in the literature. An attempt was made to summarize in one place the available evidence, and when possible to compare and point out the advantages and disadvantages of different techniques for localization of BoNT injections. The widely applied clinical indications for dystonia and spasticity have been specifically chosen as our focus in this present work.

Keywords: dystonia, spasticity, BoNT, injection, localization, techniques

1. Introduction

Botulinum toxin (BoNT), the most potent biological toxin, has become a powerful therapeutic tool for a growing number of clinical indications. There are seven distinct serotypes of BoNT —A, B, C (C-1, C-2), D, E, F, and G—that have similar neurotoxic properties resulting in flaccid muscle paralysis due to presynaptic blockage of acetylcholine release [1]. Double-blind placebo-controlled studies, as well as open-label clinical trials, provide evidence that when appropriate targets and doses are selected, BoNT temporarily ameliorates disorders associated with excessive muscle contraction or autonomic dysfunction [2]. BoNT/A and B are the most studied serotypes, commercially available and extensively used. Today BoNT/A is employed and considered safe and effective for treatment of movement disorders, with dystonia and spasticity being the most widely used indications. The BoNT serotypes, however, differ in their intracellular protein target, potency, and duration of action. These properties differ even between preparations that contain the same BoNT serotype due to variations in product formulations [3]. Recent changes to the established drug names were intended to reinforce these differences and prevent medication errors. The products and their approved indications include the following: onabotulinumtoxin A (Botox, Botox Cosmetic)—cervical dystonia (CD), severe primary axillary hyperhidrosis, strabismus, blepharospasm, upper and lower limb spasticity, overactive bladder, urinary incontinence, and migraine headache (Food and Drug Administration (FDA)). In the European Union (EU), it was approved also for the treatment of hemifacial spasm. Abobotulinumtoxin A (Dysport)—cervical dystonia, upper limb spasticity, moderate-to-severe glabellar lines (FDA), plus blepharospasm, hemifacial spasm, hyperhidrosis, strabismus, and cerebral palsy (EU). Incobotulinumtoxin A (Xeomin) —cervical dystonia, blepharospasm, upper limb spasticity, and glabellar lines. Rimabotulinumtoxin B (Myobloc, NeuroBloc)—cervical dystonia [4].

A retrospective long-term (10 year) BoNT/B study showed that although most patients required increased dosage, BoNT/B was an effective and safe treatment for a variety of movement disorders [5]. BoNT/F has been intensively tested, but due to its short-term effect, lasting about a month, it is not widely used in clinical practice [6].

The effectiveness of BoNT treatment depends on the proper selection of indications, protein content of the formulation, frequency of applications, dose, concentration, and injecting volume. It is also critically dependent on the appropriate localization of the intended target muscle(s), producing the abnormal movement, be it dystonic or spastic [7]. However, it is necessary not only to identify the proper muscles but also to localize the injection tip in a specific muscle area, namely the motor end-plate zone. A recent study compared low-dose BoNT injections applied into the end-plate zone with those injected at fixed distances from it at the same muscle. Injections only 1 cm apart reduced the effect of BoNT by 46%. Thus, precise end-plate-targeted injections increase the effect of BoNT and may reduce the required dosage, treatment costs, and also minimize side effects such as unwanted weakness of adjacent muscles [8]. However, motor end-plate zone location is not always easy to find. In order to facilitate its targeting, some efforts have been made for establishing the localization of the end-plate zone in different muscles in reference to external anatomical landmarks [9–11]. Another phenomenon that should be kept in mind is the diffusion of the toxin, after injection, because it may be a reason for the weakness of adjacent uninjected muscles. Diffusion may be influenced by the BoNT serotype and occur in direct proportion to the concentration of BoNT. Small size of target muscle and increased distance of needle tip from the neuromuscular junction can also result in increased diffusion of BoNT locally. This diffusion may be advantageous, however, when injecting muscles in children who may not be able to tolerate the pain associated with attempts to target the muscle. On the other hand, when treating dystonia or spasticity, diffusion of BoNT is clearly undesirable [12]. As BoNT diffusion correlates with dose, it once again favours injecting into the motor end-plate zone where administering a lower dose of the toxin provides satisfactory disease control with the possibility for less side effects. Not only higher doses but also the administration of injections in intervals shorter than 3 months is associated with the development of BoNT antibodies, leading to resistance to the specific BoNT serotype used [13]. Thus, there is a general consensus among experts that selection of the appropriate muscle and subsequent injection of the optimal dose are the most important determinants of the outcome of BoNT treatment [14].

A literature review was performed in order to summarize, and when possible, to compare and point out the advantages and disadvantages of different techniques for localization of BoNT injection. Revised techniques comprised clinically established specific sites of injecting commonly affected muscles in focal dystonia and spasticity, as well as several techniques facilitating the injection accuracy including electromyography (EMG): passive EMG (EMG guidance; EMG monitoring) and active EMG guidance (electrical stimulation), imaging, or endoscopic guidance.

2. Dystonia

Dystonia is a movement disorder characterized by sustained or intermittent muscle contractions that cause twisting and repetitive movements, abnormal postures, or both. It results from involuntary concomitant contraction of agonist and antagonist muscles, with overflow of unwanted muscle contractions into adjacent muscles. Dystonia may be clinically classified according to its distribution as focal dystonia (affecting a single body part in isolation), segmental dystonia, hemidystonia, and generalized dystonia [15]. Primary dystonia is the most common type and primary focal dystonia is 10 times as common as primary generalized torsion dystonia. Primary focal dystonia occurs nearly always in adults and may involve the neck, face, or arm, whereas the leg is rarely involved [16].

Localized BoNT injections provide a symptomatic relief in primary and non-primary dystonia syndromes, as demonstrated by several randomized controlled trials and by a large number of uncontrolled studies. BoNT is the first-choice treatment for most types of focal dystonia and could be an effective treatment option for some segmental forms. The effect begins usually about a week after injections and lasts for about 3 months [4, 17].

2.1. Blepharospasm

Blepharospasm is the second most common form of focal dystonia. Blepharospasm describes dystonia in the orbicularis oculi and, optionally, its adjacent muscles, including the corrugator supercilii, procerus, nasalis, and levator labii superioris alaeque nasi muscles [7]. It usually affects both eyes and is characterized by noticeably increased frequency of blink rate, enduring spasms of eyelids. It could significantly impair the voluntary eyelid opening which, in extreme cases, may render the patient functionally blind [18].

BoNT therapy is the treatment of choice for blepharospasm with a 90% efficacy rate of BoNT/A injections and is also safe during long-term treatment [19–23]. Evidence supported a Level A recommendation for BoNT/A, A/Inco, and A/Ona; a Level B recommendation for A/Abo; and a Level U recommendation for B/Rima [17, 24]. Adverse events include ptosis, tearing, blurred vision, double vision, dry eyes, and facial weakness [25]. Distant side effects are dose dependent and likely a result of toxin entering the circulatory or lymphatic system. Therefore, delivering the least effective amount of toxin in the most accurate manner decreases the risk of unwanted local and distant side effects as well as the risk of the development of neutralizing antibodies [23, 26, 27].

2.1.1. Anatomic/clinical muscle selection and localization of the injection needle

Although the beneficial effects of BoNT/A are self-evident, there are still several unresolved problems, referred to the optimal injection sites of BoNT [28].

The orbicularis oculi muscle consists of three portions: orbital portion, surrounding the orbital margin, including the brow, palpebral, and pretarsal portion [7]. The orbicularis oculi muscles lie immediately beneath the skin, and it is recommended that there is no need of EMG control during BoNT application [26, 29–31]. The muscle is readily accessible with a 27-, 30-, or 32-gauge needle [26, 30, 32]. Subcutaneous injections will readily spread into the underlying orbicularis muscle. A highly recommended injection strategy is the application of two injections into the upper lid near the canthus medially and laterally in order to avoid the bulk of the levator palpebrae muscle and consequent ptosis. Two lower lid injections are applied to the middle portion and to the lower lateral canthus, respectively. Avoiding the medial canthus spares the nasolacrimal apparatus [33]. A prospective trial compared four different patterns of injection sites: standard (medial and lateral aspects of the upper eyelid, and lateral and central portion of the lower eyelid), brow, inner orbital, and outer orbital. The inner orbital treatment produced significantly more episodes of ptosis (13%) and the standard the highest rate of epiphora and ocular irritation (18%). Thus, the further away from the eyelid margin the injection was, the lower risk of ocular side effects occurred [34]. Other studies summarized that the orbital portion of the orbicularis muscle should be injected at three to six sites peripherally to the orbital rim [30] and the periocular region might be injected at five to eight sites, depending on the severity and duration of the problem [35]. Mimic muscles adjacent to the orbicularis oculi, such as the procerus, the corrugator supercilii, and the nasalis muscles, may also be used as target muscles [7, 26].

Data of more special interest suggested that BoNT injections into the pretarsal portion of orbicularis oculi muscles increased the magnitude of the therapeutic response and decreased the number of unsuccessful treatments and ptosis [18, 32]. Aramideh et al. (1995) compared the response to BoNT/A according to a triple injection technique (two injections into the upper eyelid and one injection into the lower eyelid) and injections additionally applied into the pretarsal portion. The number of successful treatments with the additional pretarsal injections increased significantly from 81% to 95%, and ptosis occurred significantly less often [28].

http://dx.doi.org/10.5772/64218

Another study also confirmed the superior efficacy of pretarsal rather than orbital injections in 49 primary and secondary non-responders with blepharospasm [36]. A controlled study of 32 [37] and another study of 25 patients with blepharospasm [38] also revealed that pretarsal injections rather than preseptal injections were associated with better efficacy and significantly less ptosis. In 10 blepharospasm patients treated unsuccessfully with conventional bilateral periorbital injections, injecting BoNT into the pretarsal region proved to be highly effective, while the amount of toxin used was considerably less than that used in conventional methods [39].

2.1.2. Electromyography-controlled BoNT applications

Although EMG examination is not a routine strategy for localization of the injections [31, 32], a number of studies used EMG as a guide for accuracy in injecting BoNT into different portions of orbicularis oculi and in some other facial muscles [23, 28].

Besides, EMG studies of the levator palpebrae and orbicularis oculi muscles are instrumental in improving the understanding of the variable responses to BoNT application [26, 40, 41].

2.2. Oromandibular dystonia

Phenomenologically, there are seven types of oromandibular dystonia (OMD): jaw-closing dystonia (JCD), jaw-opening dystonia (JOD), jaw-deviation dystonia (JDD), lip and perioral dystonia, lingual dystonia, pharyngeal dystonia, and combinations. Most of the patients suffer from JCD [42]. Associated features may include protrusion or twisting of the tongue, as well as the involvement of facial, neck, and pharyngeal muscles [7].

OMD responds poorly to systemic therapy, yet a number of small open-label trials indicated significant improvement with BoNT/A injection [18]. Patients with JCD have a better response on BoNT therapy than patients with the other types of movements (JOD or JDD) [43]. JCD injections include the masseters and the temporal muscles; medial pterygoids may also be targeted. In JOD, the focus should be primarily on the lateral pterygoids. The submentalis complex (mylohyoid, geniohyoid, and anterior digastric muscles) has been targeted as well [33].

Palpation may be a helpful approach, but not all muscles are palpable. Another strategy may be to monitor muscle activity by EMG (passive EMG guidance) and inject those that showed increased activity during the particular abnormal movement or posture. However, this is not always possible because EMG recordings of all involved muscles during action dystonia, such as OMD, are technically difficult [42].

2.2.1. Anatomic/clinical muscle selection and localization of the injection needle

In a prospective study of 162 patients, the muscle selection was based on clinical observation and examination coupled with extensive, long-term experience. The masseters and submental muscles were injected with BoNT/A. With a moderate-to-marked improvement, responded 80% of the JCD; 40% of JOD, 33% of JDD, and 52% of the combinations. Complications such as dysphagia and dysarthria were reported in 19% of the JCD and in 40% of the JOD patients. There was a poorer response and higher complication rate in the JOD than in the JCD [43]. Later on, the study group has modified its technique by directing the injection needle into the most anterior portion of the submental complex and administering the total dosage as a single bolus, which resulted in a marked reduction in dysphagia and other complications [42].

2.2.2. Electromyography-controlled BoNT applications

Brin et al. (1994) described their experience with 96 patients with OMD. Muscle selection was made using EMG and a relatively large number of muscles were considered for injection. EMG was always used to inject the pterygoids (preferentially the external pterygoids) and usually to inject the other muscles. If necessary, the digastrics and submentals were also injected. In all movement categories, patients' function improved from about 30% of normal function to about 74%. Adverse effects were seen in 14% of the patients. Only one case of dysphagia was severe enough to require a change in diet. Most cases of dysphagia were seen in the patients with JOD and were associated with injection of the digastrics [42, 44]. Because of different methods of muscle selection and different injection techniques (clinical and EMG) used by Tan et al. (1999) and Brin et al. (1994), as well as different methods of assessing severity, response, and adverse effects, it is impossible to compare the two studies; the overall results, however, appeared to be similar [42].

An open-label BoNT/A treatment trial of X-linked dystonia-parkinsonism reported 50 cases of OMD and 35 cases of lingual dystonia to be injected under EMG guidance. The OMD group included 32 cases with JOD, 12 cases with JCD, and 6 cases with JDD. The lingual dystonia group consisted of 27 cases with tongue protrusion and 8 cases with tongue curling. All the OMD types as well as lingual dystonias showed substantial improvement at week 4. Adverse events occurred in 19% of the JOD and in 17% of the JCD patients, as the most frequent of them were mouth dryness and dysphagia. The investigators observed higher rate of mouth dryness, particularly with percutaneous lateral pterygoid injections. On the other hand, they stated an opinion that the lateral pterygoid should be injected, as it was a major force producer in JOD, and the treated dystonia was severe, with associated pain. The bilateral intraoral approach under EMG guidance appeared to be safer, faster, and more convenient, rather than the percutaneous approach when treating JOD. The most common adverse event during the lingual dystonia treatment was dysphagia, which occurred in 19% of the tongue protrusion and in 13% of the tongue curling cases [45].

A study evaluated 45 patients treated with quantitative EMG-guided injections of BoNT for OMD: 11 patients with JCD, 7 with JOD, and 13 patients with OMD of mixed type. Marked effect was observed in 70% of the cases. Side effects occurred in 35.6%, most frequently as transient mild dysphagia, thus indicating quantitative EMG BoNT treatment was safe and effective [46]. A report of four cases with OMD that involved the lateral pterygoid muscles producing incapacitating protrusive and lateral jaw movements and displacements used graphic assessment of jaw movements by a magnetic tracking system. The EMG activity was recorded by needle electrodes applying an intraoral approach, whereas the activity of masseter muscles was recorded with surface electrodes. EMG-guided BoNT injections into the muscles

http://dx.doi.org/10.5772/64218

led to marked reduction of the OMD severity, the mandibular movements, and the functional disturbances [47].

In general, the use of EMG has been suggested for muscles that are not superficially palpable, but it has not been validated [18]. Recently, some authors recommend all injections for OMD to be complemented with EMG guidance and performed with a hollow, 27-gauge, Teflon-coated, monopolar needle. To minimize the risk of contamination, the intraoral injections should be administered last [30, 48]. Other authors indicated that pterygoid muscle injections have to be performed with EMG guidance, as the muscles are not easily accessible to palpation. The EMG-guided approach was often helpful for other jaw muscles, such as the digastric, masseter, and temporalis [4].

In some forms of lingual dystonia, as with the case of tongue protrusion dystonia, because of the various muscles involved in tongue protrusion, as well as jaw opening, they could not be reliably differentiated either clinically or by EMG sampling. This, however, did not hamper the good results from BoNT injections in the 'submental muscles', although some swallowing difficulties could be triggered [42]. There are still unresolved issues concerning the best method of identifying and selectively injecting the most appropriate muscles, as well as the importance of EMG or ultrasound (US) in this process [42].

2.2.3. *Ultrasound-guided BoNT injections*

In 46 patients with temporomandibular disorders, the anterior temporalis, anterior masseter, deep masseter, anterior digastric, posterior digastric, and sternocleidomastoid muscles were measured bilaterally by US with satisfactory visualization [49]. In clinical practice, however, US guidance is not feasible for the pterygoid muscles and is only hardly feasible for the mimic and pharyngeal muscles, probably because of their direct accessibility. Supra- and infrahyoid as well as temporalis and masseter muscles can be visualized with US. However, guided BoNT injection in this area is rarely necessary [50, 51].

2.3. Laryngeal dystonia (adductor and abductor spasmodic dystonia)

Spasmodic dysphonia (SD) is a rare form of focal dystonia—laryngeal dystonia [52]. It results in irregular, uncontrolled contraction of the laryngeal musculature during phonation. SD is task specific and typically affects connected speech. It can be subdivided, based on the clinical signs and symptoms, into adductor, abductor, or mixed types [53].

The adductor type, caused by spasmodic activity of the vocal muscle (thyroarytenoid), is the most common type affecting 80–90% of SD patients. It induces hyperadduction of the vocal folds during speaking, producing a voice that is harsh, often tremulous, with inappropriate pitch or pitch breaks, breathiness, and glottal fry [4, 54]. The abductor, a less common type, is due to spasms of the posterior cricoarytenoid muscles (PCA), causing a prolonged, inappropriate abduction of vocal folds during voiceless consonants. This results in a breathy, effortful, hypophonic voice with abrupt termination of voicing and aphonic or whispered segments of speech [4].

BoNT/A, or BoNT/B, if there is resistance to type A, is considered the first-line treatment for SD [55]. Most investigators report a 75–95% improvement in voice symptoms and in quality of life [4, 56]. Adverse events include transient breathy hypophonia, hoarseness and occasional dysphagia, dyspnea, and stridor [57].

For adductor SD, the preferred treatment modality is the injection of BoNT into the intrinsic adductor muscle compartment of the larynx that includes most often the thyroarytenoid and, if a satisfactory effect was not observed, the lateral cricoarytenoid muscle as well [58]. Hillel et al. (2004) suggested that interarytenoid muscle may be an active dystonic muscle and should be treated in selected patients [59]. Treatment of abductor SD is challenging, because BoNT injections into the PCA often results in only partial symptom relief. This may be due to inaccurate placement into PCA. Meleca et al. (1997) described a transcricoid technique and compared it with the standard retrocricoid approach in six patients. Both practitioners and patients preferred the transcricoid method because of less discomfort, equivalent or better voice results, and fewer side effects [57, 60]. For treating abductor SD, the cricothyroid muscle can also be injected [4].

Unilateral or bilateral protocols have been proposed for treating both SD types [4, 61]. There are a variety of injection approaches to deliver BoNT into the intrinsic laryngeal adductor compartment, including EMG guidance, the 'point-touch' technique, a transnasal or transoral approach, and percutaneous fiberscopic guidance. No particular technique has been shown to be superior to another [53, 62].

2.3.1. Anatomic/clinical muscle selection and localization of the injection needle

The 'point-touch' technique is an injection method which relies on anatomical landmarks. It is cheaper, quicker and more accessible, but has not yet gained widespread acceptance due to concerns about patient satisfaction. In a prospective study of 37 patients with adductor SD, post-treatment results showed significantly improved swallowing [63]. A retrospective study compared the effectiveness of BoNT injection between EMG-guided and 'point-touch' techniques in the treatment of adductor SD for a period of 8 years. No endoscopic guidance or verification was utilized for injections using the 'point-touch' technique, as based purely on externally palpable laryngeal landmarks. Using a 1.5-inch 27-gauge needle, BoNT was introduced percutaneously into the laryngeal adductor compartment. Adequate needle positioning was guided by palpation and external landmark visualization alone. By the EMG-guided method a 37-mm 27-gauge monopolar, hollow-bore, Teflon-coated EMG needle was inserted percutaneously into the area of the thyroarytenoid muscle with the most active motor unit action potentials (MUAPs). There were no statistically significant differences in the rate of effective injections (94.4 and 93.2%, respectively; $p = 0.7$), need to alter dose, breathiness, or dysphagia. These results suggested that the BoNT treatment efficacy depends not only on the injection method used but also on the experience of the physician [53]. It seemed that the 'point-touch' technique can be well tolerated by the patient. But it is a true blind technique and visualization of the vocal folds may be required to confirm accurate placement of the needle tip in the thyroarytenoid muscle [62]. Another version of the 'point-touch' technique actually represented an anatomic approach to BoNT injection that requires only a flexible nasophar-

http://dx.doi.org/10.5772/64218

yngeal endoscopy and careful evaluation of the anatomic landmarks. This technique has been used successfully by Green et al. (1992) on 13 patients with adductor SD [64].

2.3.2. Electromyography-controlled BoNT applications

Experienced clinicians suggested that there are several unique instances in which needle EMG guidance is necessary to achieve optimal results and avoid side-effects, and one of them is the percutaneous BoNT injections into vocal cords for the treatment of SD [14, 32]. It was even thought to be the 'gold standard' for adductor SD treatment [63]. In a double-blind treatment trial of BoNT versus saline, laryngeal EMG-guided injections into the thyroarytenoid muscle were beneficial [65]. Several studies confirmed that BoNT transcutaneous injections under EMG control into thyroarytenoid muscle represented a safe and effective treatment strategy [64, 66]. The results obtained, however, did not suggest inferiority of other techniques of non-EMG guided laryngeal BoNT delivery [53]. In a retrospective study of 25 patients with adductor SD, treated with EMG-guided BoNT injection into the thyroarytenoid muscle, substantial symptom relief was reported. However, a high percentage of side effects were observed, although transient and mild — breathiness (68%) and choking on fluid (56%) [54]. Based on the evidence, laryngeal EMG was recommended as possibly effective for the injection of BoNT into the thyroarytenoid muscle in the treatment of adductor SD [65]. A relative drawback of the method might be the need for EMG confirmation of needle placement [64].

EMG-guided BoNT injections are also used as a treating method in abductor type of SD. Blitzer et al. (1992) reported 32 patients who have been treated by sequential percutaneous EMG-guided injections of the PCA muscles and improved to an average of 70% of normal voice. Ten patients, however, required injection of the cricothyroid muscles and type I laryngoplasty [67]. A prospective randomized crossover trial compared two injection techniques—via either a percutaneous posterior-lateral approach (with EMG-guidance) or an endoscopic (transnasal fiberoptic) approach. Although patients perceived some benefits, blinded symptom counts did not substantiate significant reductions in the numbers of breathy breaks occurred with either techniques, and no differences were found between both techniques. Thus, BoNT/A injections into PCA muscle provided limited benefits to patients with abductor SD, demonstrating the need of a more effective therapy [68].

An advantage of EMG guidance is the confirmation of needle's placement within the muscles of the larynx by showing distinct MUAP with phonation, thus ensuring delivery of the exotoxin into the most active portion of the muscle, near the motor end plate [62]. Using a non-EMG-guided technique, placement of the needle into the vicinity of the muscle can be achieved, but it is not possible to confirm placement into the most active portion of the muscle. It is questionable whether BoNT needs to be delivered to the electrically most active portion, or if the EMG signal is just an aid to direct the needle into the correct muscle. On the one hand, it is assumed that more accurately placed dose in a particular muscle should reduce any side effects in an adjacent muscle. On the other hand, it has been demonstrated that BoNT easily passes through muscle fascia and can disseminate to the nearby muscles. It may be that once the needle is in the vicinity of the correct muscle, toxin delivered will dose the entire muscle regardless of needle tip proximity to the most active MUAP [53]. Some authors state that injecting by EMG guidance is more precise and uses the lowest therapeutic dose [69]. Cited disadvantages include the possibility that EMG signal may be misleading, and the technique is more time consuming, redundant to anatomic localization, or even more uncomfortable due to additional needle positioning and manoeuvring. A few minor disadvantages to laryngeal EMG-guided BoNT administration may be related to a greater patient discomfort due to an inherent longer period of needle placement during the search for MUAPs [53]. Some authors suppose, however, that percutaneous injection with laryngoscopic guidance is less precise [69], although there is not clear evidence to support the superiority of any particular localization technique.

2.3.3. Endoscopy control

Although BoNT injection under EMG guidance is the standard for the thyroarytenoid muscle, in some instances, endoscopy-controlled BoNT placement could be an alternative [62]. Klap et al. (1991) reported satisfactory effect of direct BoNT injections into the thyroarytenoid muscle under fiberoptic visualization in six patients, followed for a period of 2 years [52]. In a retrospective study, a total of 426 BoNT injections were administered in 64 adductor CD patients under laryngoscopy guidance with satisfactory results, especially when BoNT injection was placed at the posterior portion of the thyroarytenoid and directed towards the lateral cricoarytenoid so that both muscle groups were affected [61]. A retrospective open trial investigated the effect of toxin preparation and injection monitoring on 15 patients with adductor SD. BoNT was administered into the vocalis muscle by 112 and 36 injections under EMG or laryngoscopy guidance, respectively. Failure rate did not differ, using EMG (28.6%) or laryngoscopy (30.5%) guidance. The treatment failure may occur regardless of the method of injection, possibly due to mislocalization of the vocal folds [70]. Thirty patients with adductor SD were randomly allocated into an EMG or a fiberscopy-guided BoNT treatment group. There were no significant differences in outcomes between the two groups in either the duration of effectiveness or complications such as breathy voice and aspiration. BoNT injection under fiberscopy guidance appeared to be a valuable alternative to EMG-guided treatment in adductor SD. The fiberscopy-guided percutaneous injections have demonstrated high reliability of confirming needle location. A source of discomfort may be the need of local anaesthesia to aid the insertion of the fiberscope [62]. There is, however, limited number of studies, comparing the endoscope-controlled injection placement with other guidance techniques, and additional investigations have to be performed in the field.

2.3.4. Ultrasound-guided BoNT injection

In laryngeal muscles, US guidance is hardly feasible. The laryngeal muscles (vocalis, PCA) can be injected transorally using endoscopic guidance, or transdermally. For transdermal injection, EMG guidance is crucial, either alone or, optionally, in combination with US [50].

2.4. Cervical dystonia

CD is the most common form of focal dystonia and is marked by deviation of the head around horizontal (torticollis), coronal (retrocollis, anterocollis), and vertical axis (laterocollis), often associated with reduced range of motion in the direction contralateral to the movement. Horizontal rotation is the most common abnormal movement, affecting 80% of the patients. It typically arises from activity of the sternocleidomastoid muscle contralateral to the turn and splenius capitis muscle ipsilateral to the direction of turn. Deeper muscles, including the longissimus capitis, splenius cervices, longus capitis, and obliquus capitis, can also be involved. Laterocollis is seen in 10–20% and ipsilateral splenius, sternocleidomastoid, and levator scapulae muscles are involved. Retrocollis and anterocollis are less frequent and involve bilateral posterior and anterior muscles, respectively. Often combinations of torticollis and laterocollis are presented. Shoulder involvement is present in approximately half of the patients. Associated pain is reported in 70–75% [7].

BoNT is the first-line treatment of idiopathic CD, and all commercially available BoNT brands have proven satisfactory symptom relief in more than 85% of the cases [22, 32, 71]. Adverse events are generally mild or moderate and transient, including pain at injection site, neck weakness, flu-like symptoms, hoarseness, dry mouth, and dysphagia. Systemic events include general fatigue and muscle weakness [4].

The most injected muscles are the sternocleidomastoid, splenius capitis, trapezius descendens/semispinalis capitis, trapezius horizontalis, levator scapulae, scalenii, and deep neck muscles [30, 50].

2.4.1. *Anatomic/clinical muscle selection and localization of the injection needle*

In the large and easily accessible muscles, typically treated in CD, clinical placement seems sufficient for the majority of patients [30, 32]. On physical examination, muscles should be palpated for hypertrophy, activity and contracture, or fibrosis. Areas of pain should be noted [30], as BoNT alleviates pain as well [72]. Manual application into the upper third of the sternocleidomastoid muscle is often sufficient to reduce dysphagia considerably [50].

2.4.2. *Electromyography-controlled BoNT applications*

The majority of electrophysiological techniques applied for BoNT treatment of CD implied polymiographic EMG for muscle detection and guidance of the injection needle [73]. Electric stimulation (ES) is considered not to be feasible because the response of neck muscles to the stimulus is not specific enough [74]. Only few EMG frequency analysis studies, with limited number of patients enrolled, are advocating some benefits in targeting more specifically the leading dystonic muscles [73]. The need of EMG guidance for CD patients remains an issue of controversy [26]. Although superficial muscles that may be readily palpated are usually involved, Barbano (2001) suggested that needle EMG exploration of the dystonic neck often revealed affecting of deeper muscles which are difficult to access. Furthermore, muscles with opposing actions are often in close proximity, making it possible to do more harm than good with poorly targeted injections [75]. Several studies reported benefits of EMG-guided BoNT injections. Speelman and Brans (1995) showed the benefits of EMG guidance when the accuracy of sternocleidomastoid localization in 139 EMG-guided injections was examined. They found that 83% of needle placement attempts reached the target muscles [76]. According to Wulff et al. (1993), the EMG guidance proved to be helpful as it restricted the injections into muscles with EMG hyperactivity, thereby economizing the amount of toxin given. They conducted a study of 20 idiopathic torticollis patients, who received EMG-guided intramuscular BoNT/A injections. An overall improvement of 55%, in comparison to the status before treatment was found, and side effects were restricted to short-term dysphagia in two patients [77]. Based on the results of 84 patients, receiving injection under EMG guidance, Dubinsky et al. (1991) revealed treatment effectiveness in 78.7%. The complications included excessive neck weakness, which was observed in 16.0% and dysphagia—presented in 11.1% of the injection sessions [78]. Comella et al. (1992) randomized 52 CD patients into two groups. In the first one, both clinical and needle EMG examinations were used for muscle selection, and injections were performed by EMG assistance. In the second group, muscle selection was based solely on the clinical examination and manual needle location. The EMG assistance did not increase the number of patients improved, but the magnitude of improvement was significantly greater. Moreover, in particular patients with retrocollis, head tilt, and shoulder elevation, additional benefit with EMG-guided BoNT injection were noted [79]. In a prospective study, Lee et al. (2004) evaluated 15 CD patients. In those who underwent EMG-guided BoNT injection, there were fewer BoNT-related side effects due to injection of the adequate dose to the accurate site of hyperactive muscles. Besides, a greater clinical improvement due to confirmation of hyperactivity in target muscles and a better ability to reduce the amount of oral medication were reported. EMG-guided BoNT injections were considered to be useful for patients with retrocollis, for those who have had a suboptimal treatment response to non EMG-guided BoNT injections, and for those with increased concern of side effects or a concomitant goal of reducing oral medications [80]. In a recent, one-year prospective, randomized, and blinded study, Werdelin et al. (2011) evaluated 20 CD patients, comparing EMG-guided injections with chemodenervation after clinical evaluation alone. Quantitative EMG was performed simultaneously in the sternocleidomastoid muscles and the posterior neck muscles on both sides. In patients treated on EMG guidance, clinical outcome, evaluated by objective ratings, was better than in patients treated on clinical judgement alone. In a group blinded, 105 muscles were injected with BoNT, but 37 of those did not show dystonic EMG activity. EMG guidance by interference pattern analysis appeared to optimize BoNT treatment by more precise injection localization and may reduce the amount of the toxin used, side effects, and the risk of development of antibodies [81].

Although the advantages of EMG-guided BoNT application were reported, in most studies, EMG was used not only for injection guidance but also for muscle selection. Due to that reason, some authors advised that all these studies should be interpreted with caution [74]. A recent review, focused on identifying the best method for muscle selection in CD patients, compared EMG techniques with clinical examination and revealed that EMG-guided injections may improve the treatment outcome but did not show an overall better outcome compared to clinical muscle selection and anatomical needle placement [73]. In the presented pooled analysis of 28 studies of which 17 used clinical evaluation to identify dystonic muscles and 11 used EMG for selection and guidance, better results for the EMG approach regarding pain reduction (−40.3 vs.−32.5 %) were recorded. However, improvement was lower for EMG compared to clinical evaluation by rating scales like the Tsui score (−31.9 vs.−43.7%) [73].

Some critical remarks also question the superiority of EMG-guided injections in routine treatment of CD. It has to be taken into account that positioning of the EMG needle is performed according to anatomic landmarks. The placement of the EMG needle tip into a specific muscle is thereby almost impossible to verify, as selective voluntary activation of neck muscles is not possible and might be additionally superimposed by dystonic activity of adjacent muscles. EMG therefore serves more as a 'functional' guidance than as an anatomical guidance. The assignment of EMG activity to specific muscles is flawed by the same anatomic inaccuracy as needle placement according to anatomical landmarks. Searching for dystonic EMG activity is associated with additional discomfort and pain for the patients. It is more time-consuming and requires some extra costs [74]. Besides, needle EMG does not differentiate between contractions produced by agonist versus antagonist muscles and may be misleading if the patient 'tenses' uninvolved muscles. If a muscle is obviously contracting or is hypertrophied, needle EMG is redundant. A strong argument implies that if the results of BoNT treatment without needle EMG are good, a small additional improvement does not justify the routine use of EMG [14].

On the other hand, based on clinical experience and an investigation of 20 CD cases, Cordivari et al. (2006) suggested that if a patient started to respond poorly to BoNT/A and resistance to the product was excluded, a re-examination and careful placement of injections under EMG guidance may improve the treatment outcome [82].

According to the Therapeutics and Technology Assessment Subcommittee of the American Academy of Neurology, the role of EMG has not been established for CD [17]. It may contribute for improving the outcome, especially in complex forms [32] or in secondary non-responders [82]. Still, evidence is limited and larger studies are needed [73].

2.4.3. *Ultrasound-guided BoNT injections*

Although BoNT/A has a favourable safety profile and is effective in the majority of patients with CD, in some cases, the treatment outcome is disappointing or side effects occur when higher doses are used. It is likely that in such cases either the target muscles were not injected accurately or unintended weakness of non-target muscles occurred [74]. Mezaki et al. (2000) described an US investigation of cervical muscles for 20 dystonic patients compared with healthy controls. They found contracting synergists responsible for the abnormal posture, a finding not presented in healthy controls. The investigators suggested US to be an accurate method for localizing the contracting muscles during injection, although the treating substance used was not BoNT, but lidocaine and pure ethanol [83]. US is of special value as the injected muscles differ in size, and the deep-seated muscles require a different approach compared to superficial ones [74]. Besides being a useful guidance, Mezaki (2011) suggested that it may be even superior to the EMG monitoring, especially when the obliquus capitis inferior muscle is targeted in rotatocollis, because the vertebral artery or upper cervical nerve root(s) may be injured when the needle penetrates the muscle [72]. Dysphagia is a common side effect after BoNT injections for CD, with an incidence of 10–40%, depending upon the study and dose used. Hong et al. (2012) examined the effects on swallowing using EMG guidance for BoNT injection and dysphagia occurred in 34.7%. Using US, combined with EMG guidance, there was no dysphagia across 27 injection sessions, possibly because of retaining the injected toxin within the muscle [84]. Schramm et al. (2015) recently conducted a review of the relevance of sonography in CD and provided a statement from clinical experts for its use. In the authors' opinion, the routine use of US injection guidance could be recommended in general, as it facilitates anatomically precise and reproducible injections in specific muscles. Ordinary injected muscles are the splenius capitis, sternocleidomastoideus, semispinalis capitis, and levator scapulae muscles, as well as more difficult accessible, small, or deeply located muscles like the longus colli, longus capitis, scalene, and obliquus capitis inferior and superior muscles. This method might prevent unintended muscle weakness due to diffusion of BoNT, bearing in mind that injected neck muscles may be small or thin and lie in close proximity to each other. US is also indispensable when case-specific anatomic conditions are present such as obesity or very pronounced neck muscles, or even muscle atrophy, occurring in consequence of previous treatments. Furthermore, US helps in preventing injection in blood vessels and nerves. This might be of special importance in CD as injections in lateral cervical muscles bear a high risk for injuries of adjacent structures (carotid artery, thyroid truncus, internal and external jugular vein, vagal nerve, phrenic nerve, and brachial plexus). With injections in the dorsal neck region, the vertebral artery or the spinal canal may be erroneously injected. Moreover, US guidance offers the potential for dose reduction. That may decrease the risk of producing neutralizing antibodies and therefore ensure long-term efficacy of treatment. The combination of US and EMG could overcome the shortcomings of EMG regarding anatomic precision and would allow an accurate assignment of dystonic activity to specific muscles [74]. However, as there are only a few small randomized studies suggesting superiority of sonography guidance compared to conventional needle placement, US guidance should be investigated in future clinical studies [50].

2.4.4. Positron emission tomography/computer tomography control

Herting et al. (2004) reported a case of a patient, suffering from severe anterocollis, where repeated computer tomography (CT)-controlled injections of BoNT into the right longus colli muscle allowed a precise location of the needle and injection of the toxin, leading to an obvious improvement of symptoms [85].

As it is well known that glucose metabolism and 18F-FDG uptake are enhanced in contracting skeletal muscles, it was suggested that the degree of 18F-FDG uptake may be associated with the strength of contraction. Moreover, an integrated positron emission tomography/computer tomography (PET/CT) controlled method was found to provide both metabolic and anatomic information on hypermetabolic lesions [86, 87]. Sung et al. (2007) investigated six patients with idiopathic CD. BoNT injections into target muscles were performed with Teflon-coated monopolar needle electrode cannula guided by EMG. For deep cervical muscles adjacent to a major artery or the major nerve trunk (obliquus capitis inferior and longus colli muscles), BoNT was injected under CT or US guidance. All four patients who underwent PET/CT-guided injections experienced a significant improvement in symptoms, even though in three of these patients, previous BoNT therapy guided by clinical findings had failed [87]. Similar results were obtained by Lee et al. (2009), who conducted a study with 14 BoNT treated CD patients and compared different localization techniques. Muscles for BoNT injection were selected after considering abnormal posture type and EMG, and PET/CT findings. When selected muscles were located beyond the expected coverage of the EMG needle, near an important structure, imaging-guided injection was considered. A total of 13 BoNT injections in eight patients were performed under imaging guidance, and technical success was achieved in all cases. For injections into the longus colli muscle (poor sonic window due to the pharynx), the obliquus capitis inferior muscle, and the scalenus anterior, scalenus posterior, and levator scapulae muscles, CT guidance was chosen. Otherwise, US guidance was preferred because of its convenience. The results obtained using PET/CT and imaging guidance were superior to results obtained on the basis of physical examination or EMG [71]. Although CT provides a precise visualization of deep muscles of the neck and the surrounding structures, a disadvantage of the method is that its use is limited to a clinical setting where CT is accessible. Therefore, the use of CT has been recorded in a small number of patients. Moreover, CT is too expensive for frequent use in daily practice, it is not dynamic, and patients are exposed to radiation [50, 74].

PET has been used in two studies (mentioned above) to identify hypermetabolic and presumably dystonic muscles, whereas injection was performed under CT or US guidance [71, 87]. PET, therefore, rather represents a diagnostic method and not a method for injection control [74].

2.4.5. *Fluoroscopy (electromyography combined with fluoroscopy)*

While BoNT is the treatment of choice for CD, patients with anterocollis, who receive injections into the sternocleidomastoid and anterior scalene muscles, present a disproportionate number of treatment failures. Incomplete muscle selection may be one cause of treatment failures in anterocollis. Deep cervical muscles, such as the longus colli, are not routinely injected. Glass et al. (2009) described a technique for longus colli injection in three cases of anterocollis and reported the clinical outcomes of 10 such BoNT injections. The patients had previous treatment failures with sternocleidomastoid/anterior scalene injections or no activity was recorded during the needle EMG investigation of these muscles. All patients were injected into the longus colli under fluoroscopic and EMG guidance, which resulted in a significant symptomatic improvement (8 of 10 injections). Two patients reported mild dysphagia without serious complications after dose increased. It seems that fluoroscopic guidance allows safe and effective BoNT injections into deep cervical muscles [88]. However, fluoroscopy is associated with the application of considerable amounts of radiation and multiple intramuscular injections of iodinated contrast media, both of which can be potentially harmful [50].

2.4.6. *Magnetic resonance imaging control*

Magnetic resonance imaging (MRI) allows high-definition visualization of deep muscles, such as the longus colli and obliquus capitis inferior, glandular tissue and critical structures. Mixtures of BoNT and contrast medium allow documentation of the toxin placement. However, the visualization is not in real time, so that the relationship between the injection needle and the target tissue cannot be monitored continuously. Other disadvantages including costs and time prevent the routine use of this method [50].

2.5. Limb dystonia

Focal upper limb dystonia usually starts in the hand and is task specific; however, with progression, task specificity is gradually lost [89]. Other occupational hand dystonia and nontask-specific (fixed) dystonia are presented mainly by writer's cramp [17]. The upper extremity is affected more commonly than the lower, and most BoNT studies deal with the upper limb, and especially with writer's cramp [17, 18]. Writer's cramp is a task-specific dystonia characterized by involuntary, repetitive, or sustained contractions of finger, hand, or arm muscles that occur during writing and produce abnormal postures or movements that interfere with normal handwriting [90]. Injections for writer's cramp are usually focused on finger flexors and extensors in the forearm, but wrist pronators and flexors are often involved [18].

Foot dystonia is often presented with foot inversion, toe dorsiflexion, and/or ankle plantar flexion. The injected muscles may include tibialis posterior, extensor hallucis longus, gastrocnemius, and long toe flexors. Usually the treatment requires higher dose of the neurotoxin [4].

BoNT remains the first choice treatment, as there are no effective alternative medical or well-established surgical therapies. It is recommended as probably effective for treatment of focal upper extremity limb dystonia. BoNT treatment is considered to be possibly effective for lower extremity dystonia, but the presented data are insufficient to provide a recommendation [17, 91]. Therapeutic difficulties occur due to involving the subtle tuning of many muscles. Besides, it is difficult to obtain the requested quality of voluntary movement without weakness. Pain is the symptom most frequently improved, often independently of motor function [4]. In case of neutralizing antibodies against the A toxin, the treatment with BoNT/ B or BoNT/F is a possible alternative [32, 92]. The use of BoNT to treat limb dystonia requires thoughtful technique including customization of doses and muscle selection. The first step in treatment planning is to identify the muscles most severely affected, separating out dystonic from compensatory movements. After initial inspection, EMG- or US-guided muscle selection usually allows refining the choice of targets [89].

2.5.1. Anatomic/clinical muscle selection and localization of the injection needle versus electromyography-controlled BoNT applications: passive and active electromyographic guidance

As focal hand dystonia is a complex disorder, usually involving several muscles, and many of them are deep, not easily identified by surface landmarks and not palpable on examination, their localization is often challenging [50]. In some instances, however, physicians use their knowledge on surface anatomy and clinical examination to localize the target muscles but EMG guidance may be particularly important. In a trial, 40 patients with writer's cramp were randomized in a double-blind design to BoNT or an equivalent volume of saline placebo. Injected muscles were chosen based on clinical examination, but injections were performed under EMG guidance and a significant improvement was obtained [90]. In a prospective, double-blind crossover study of 17 patients with upper and lower limb dystonia, target muscles were identified either clinically on the basis of the abnormal posture and muscle contraction or by EMG guidance. The EMG method allowed the patient to perform the task that precipitated the cramp while EMG activity was recorded. Clinical and EMG identification

http://dx.doi.org/10.5772/64218

usually correlated well, but on some occasions, muscles identified by clinical evaluation were not regarded as abnormal by EMG and vice versa. Received injections were EMG guided. Using a patient subjective scale, 82% reported benefit; however, physician rating did not reveal significant difference in the treatment outcome. The main side effect was focal weakness that emerged after 53% of BoNT injections [93]. In another placebo-controlled, double-blind, crossover trial in 20 patients with writer's cramp, muscle selection was determined by clinical examination. In eight patients, however, EMG was employed to guide selection of muscles. Twelve patients had improvement in pen control, but only four had significant improvement in writing. Focal weakness was the only adverse event and was severe enough to worsen pen control in one patient [94]. Molloy et al. (2002) compared the efficacy of EMG-guided versus non-guided injections for limb dystonia in a randomly chosen cohort of 14 consecutive patients. Only 37% of needle placement attempts reached the proper muscles in the absence of EMG guidance. Forty-seven percent were placed in an unintended muscle or fascicle and 16% were outside the muscle altogether. Individual finger fascicles of larger muscles such as flexor digitorum profundus or extensor digitorum communis were particularly difficult to isolate accurately without EMG [95]. EMG recording during the task associated with dystonia may be helpful to pinpoint muscle activation patterns [18]. Schuele et al. (2005) demonstrated benefits of EMG guidance in a study of 84 musicians with focal task-specific dystonia, treated with EMG-guided BoNT injections, where 69% of the patients experienced improvement from the injections and 36% reported a long-term benefit in their performance ability [96]. Sojer et al. (2001) even suggested that BoNT treatment of writer's cramp required EMG-guided injections in order to avoid side effects [32]. Because of the numerous small muscles located in a close proximity, some authors give priority to an active EMG muscle selection and needle localization, namely ES. It may be applied when a common muscular origin and innervation of different adjacent muscle exist, as with the extensor digitorum, flexor digitorum sublimis, and profundus. In such cases, passive EMG guidance appeared to be less useful, as it is difficult to flex or extend these digits without also causing similar movement in the adjacent ones. However, BoNT may spread to adjacent sites by diffusion, even with use of increasing target accuracy-guiding techniques [12]. Barbano (2001) also recommended ES for upper extremity dystonia, where an inappropriate toxin placement can worsen the functional outcome by weakening non-dystonic adjacent muscles, or in cases where it is important to weaken particular fascicles of individual muscles. Moreover, ES ensures the proper localization in sedated patients or in those who otherwise would have difficulty with fine motor control, such as children [75]. Due to the lack of consensus on the best way to localize muscles in the forearm for BoNT injection, Greenen et al. (1996) conducted a study comparing EMG with ES in 12 patients with the conclusion that localization by stimulation is probably at least as good as EMG. Weakness of 'non-target' muscles was present with both techniques [97]. In a critical expert review, based on long-term experience, Jankovic (2001) concluded that there are several unique instances in which needle EMG guidance is essential to achieve optimal results. These include BoNT treatment of certain task-specific dystonias, like in keyboard and string musician's cases, that are particularly difficult to treat because accurate and well-coordinated hand and finger movements are involved. However, even in patients with occupational cramps, such as dystonic writer's cramp or focal hand tremor, an injection into the forearm flexor muscles (e.g., flexor carpi radialis and flexor carpi ulnaris) could be successfully performed by using well-defined anatomic landmarks. Benefits were obtained from local BoNT injections in patients with dystonic writer's cramp that were similar to the benefits seen when using complex EMG and fine-wire electrodes to localize bursts of muscle activation during the task and by injecting the toxin through a hollow EMG needle into the belly of the most active muscle [14, 98]. Therefore, if there is a minimal increase in improvement, the routine use of the EMG-guided approach does not justify the increased discomfort, time, and expense of this method, as compared with clinical examination. Moreover, it is known that BoNT diffuses outside of the target muscles even when these muscles are localized by ES [14].

In one series of patients with upper limb dystonia, weakness of uninjected muscles, adjacent to the injected, was found in 63% of the patients which was the primary cause of a suboptimal response in 15% of them [99]. The treatment of focal limb dystonia with BoNT is challenging, particularly in achieving sufficient neuromuscular blockade to alleviate dystonic movements without causing excessive muscle weakness. While many clinicians advocate EMG or ES to optimize needle localization for injection, further data are needed to establish this recommendation [17].

2.5.2. Ultrasound-guided BoNT injections

Active EMG guidance or US guidance (or a combination of both) has been found to be most helpful when targeting the forearm muscles especially for task-related dystonia [100]. In many patients with writer's cramp, the BoNT dose could be reduced when switching from manual application to US guidance [50]. US is feasible for proximal and distal arm muscles, intrinsic hand muscles, and leg muscles. For forearm and leg muscles, US visualization may protect sensitive adjacent structures (nerves, large vessels). The usefulness of US is low, however, in shoulder, proximal arm, and superficial axial muscles, because of their size and accessibility [50].

3. Spasticity

Central nervous system disorders with upper motor neuron dysfunction often produce spasticity and hypertonia of the limb that is dependent both on velocity and on range of motion. Besides increased tone, spasticity presents typically with increased muscle stretch reflexes, muscle spasms and clonus, weakness (spastic paralysis), and impairment of voluntary movements. Spasticity may occur in diffuse or focal pathological disorders of the brain and spinal cord. In adults, spasticity results from diverse aetiologies, including stroke, traumatic brain injury, multiple sclerosis, and neoplasm involving the central nervous system. The most common cause of spasticity in children is cerebral palsy (CP) [4, 18, 101]. In the upper extremities, the shoulder adductors, elbow flexors, wrist pronators, finger, and thumb flexors are frequently involved. In the lower extremities, hip adductors, knee extensors, and ankle plantar flexors and inverters may have increased spastic tone [18].

Treatment is aimed at prevention of contractures and improved functional outcome, without worsening weakness. Non-pharmacologic treatment options often do not provide long-term relief, and systemic interventions can have intolerable side effects [102]. BoNT efficacy is better established for spasticity in the upper rather than lower limb [4, 18]. BoNT doses used in spasticity are higher than those used in other movement disorders. The treatment effect is maintained for approximately 3–5 months [4]. Adverse events are rare, often benign and of short duration, as the majority of the self-reported adverse events include local muscular weakness or fatigue [103].

Several localization techniques are available to physicians that allow identification of the selected target muscles. These methods include anatomic localization in isolation or in conjunction with EMG guidance, ES guidance, or US guidance [102].

3.1. Anatomic/clinical muscle selection and localization of the injection needle

BoNT/A injections given by manual intramuscular needle placement in the lower extremity under general anaesthesia is an established treatment and standard of care in managing spasticity in CP children [104]. Most clinicians do so using manual technique without radiologic or EMG guidance to aid needle placement [105, 106]. This procedure is usually performed by finding the largest bulk of the muscle and injecting the toxin into several sites at mid-belly [105]. In a placebo-controlled, double-blind, randomized multicentre study, Mall et al. (2006) evaluated BoNT/A effect on adductor spasticity in 61 CP children, concluding that in large and easily accessible muscles, that are typically treated in adductor spasticity, clinical placement seems sufficient for the majority of patients [107]. However, Chin et al. (2005) investigated the accuracy of the 'free hand' intramuscular needle placement guided by anatomic landmarks, palpation, and passive stretching of the muscles with ES-guided method for upper and lower limb spasticity in 226 CP children. The accuracy of manual needle placement compared with ES was acceptable only for the gastrocnemius and soleus muscles (75%). It was unacceptable for all the other muscles investigated—the hip adductors (67%), medial hamstrings (46%), tibialis posterior (11%), biceps brachii (62%), and forearm and hand muscles (13–35%). The authors recommended using ES or other guidance techniques to aid injection preciseness [106]. In a prospective study, the accuracy of manual needle placement of 272 injections in gastrocnemius muscles of 39 children with spastic CP was checked against US. The needle was accurately inserted into gastrocnemius muscles in 78.7% of the cases. Accuracy was acceptable for gastrocnemius medialis (92.6%), but not for gastrocnemius lateralis (64.7%) [108]. A randomized controlled trial compared the efficacy of BoNT/A injection guided by ES or palpation, and 2 weeks of physiotherapy, to treat spasticity of the ankle plantar flexors in 65 children with spastic CP. The ES-guided injection group plus physiotherapy showed greater improvement in the spasticity and functional performance, than the other two groups (the BoNT/A group guided by palpation injection plus physiotherapy and the physiotherapy-only group) [109]. Some critical evaluation of the largest studies applying manual needle placement in the spastic lower extremity of CP children was performed. Warnink-Kavelaars et al. (2013) pointed as a main disadvantage of the studies the lack of a standardized injection protocol, which interfered with a correct base for accurate statistical analysis. Besides, methodological methods used did not allow the calculation of positive and negative predictive values, sensitivity, and specificity, which obscured the outcome [104]. Thus, Warnink-Kavelaars et al. (2013) developed a detailed protocol for manual intramuscular needle placement checked by passive stretching and relaxing of the target muscle (PSRM). It was developed for each individual muscle injection location of the adductor brevis, adductor longus, gracilis, semimembranosus, semitendinosus, biceps femoris, rectus femoris, gastrocnemius lateralis, gastrocnemius medialis, and soleus muscles. PSRM is a rapid intramuscular needle localization technique, useful for larger muscles, especially in the lower extremity, which can be performed without sophisticated equipment. Manual intramuscular needle placement would be assessed as a PSRM-positive verification when the needle moves upon passive stretching and relaxing of the intended muscle, or a PSRM-negative verification when there is no movement or only a small straight motion of the needle upon passive stretching and relaxing of the muscle. This needle location protocol would be verified then by means of ES [104].

Several clinical trials compared the efficacy of BoNT treatment in adults with spastic upper or lower limbs, when injections were placed only by clinical and anatomic landmarks, with those guided by ES or US. Still, Childers et al. (1996) suggested researches comparing more precise localization methods for BoNT/A injections might further establish the importance of EMG guidance [110]. A very recent randomized controlled study compared manual needle placement with ES- and US-guided techniques for BoNT injection of 60 adults with arm (wrist and finger) spasticity. One month after injection, the outcome measurement instruments used revealed greater improvement in the ES group than in the manual needle placement group. Furthermore, patients improved more in the US group than in the manual needle placement group. No difference was found between the US and the ES groups. These results implied that instrumental guidance may improve the outcome of BoNT injections into the spastic forearm muscles of stroke patients [111]. Another recent controlled trial compared the three localization techniques, mentioned above, but this time for the gastrocnemius of adults with spastic equinus after stroke. Forty-seven patients were randomized into three groups, and each patient received the same dose of BoNT/A into the lateral and medial head of the gastrocnemius muscle of the affected leg. One month after injection, the modified Ashworth scale recorded greater improvement in the US group than in the manual needle placement group. The ankle passive range of motion improved better in the US group than in the ES and the manual needle placement groups. No difference was found between groups for the Tardieu scale. A superiority of the US-guided injection technique was shown and the authors concluded that it could improve the clinical outcome of BoNT injections into the gastrocnemius of adults with spastic equinus [112]. Henzel et al. (2010) also compared US localization with surface landmark localization of BoNT injection targets for forearm muscle spasticity in 18 patients. Flexor pollicis longus, flexor carpi radialis, pronator teres, and flexor digitorum superficialis were identified by these separate localization techniques. Significant differences were observed between surface and ultrasound proximodistal and lateral coordinates for several flexor muscles. It seemed that US could improve the accuracy of toxin placement and help to avoid injection into vascular and nerve structures, so that it should be considered as an adjunct for localization in patients with upper limb spasticity [113].

Schnitzler et al. (2012) evaluated the accuracy of manual needle placement in the gastrocnemius muscles guided only by anatomical landmarks and palpation. One-hundred twenty-one practitioners were evaluated. Fifty-two injections were successful (43%) and 69 failed (57%), showing a poor success rate, regardless of the injector experience. Therefore, muscle palpation and anatomical landmarks were insufficient to ensure the accuracy of BoNT/A injections, even for large, superficial muscles [114]. In clinical practice, however, clinical landmarks and palpation are still often used for injecting superficial limb muscles.

3.2. Electromyography-controlled BoNT applications

The use of EMG or the motor point stimulation method is recommended to identify muscles targeted for injection, particularly for the smaller muscles in the forearm and hand [105]. Several case series and small studies reported a satisfactory treatment outcome when identification of the target muscles in the affected hand and forearm of post-stroke adults was made by passive EMG that was used also to guide the injection needle [115–117]. However, EMG was successfully applied also in the BoNT treatment of large, superficial, as well as deep muscles in the lower extremity. Statistically significant improvement in gait parameters were noted in the treatment of 12 chronic hemiparetic patients with pronounced lower limb extensor spasticity. The soleus, tibialis posterior, and gastrocnemius muscles of the affected side were injected using a 21-gauge Teflon-coated needle, which was also used as an EMG electrode. Injections were made at two sites close to the motor point, which was identified by standard neurophysiological techniques. The toxin was injected only when either a continuous or stretch-induced EMG activity was recorded, otherwise another injection site in the vicinity was checked [118]. An open BoNT/A effectiveness study comprised 40 patients, with moderate to severe spasticity of the upper (13) or lower limbs (27) refractory to conventional physical and medical treatments. To ensure precise muscle selection, the authors localized the target muscle primarily on clinical assessment, and after that recorded muscle activity using EMG and injected targeting the middle third of the muscle belly. The initial dosage of BoNT/A varied with individual muscles and the degree of their involvement as judged clinically and as confirmed by EMG. Thirty-four patients (85%) derived worthwhile benefit, with improved limb posture and increased range of passive motion in 31, pain reduction in 28 of 31 with pain, and improved function in 16. Side effects were limited to local and usually mild discomfort from the injections (19), symptomatic local weakness (1), and local infection (1) [119].

Active EMG guidance may be applied when treating spasticity, where it is difficult to accurately target the muscle using voluntary contraction. Following injection, however, BoNT may spread to adjacent sites by diffusion, even with the use of special guidance techniques to increase the accuracy of targeting [12]. Quantitative EMG criterion (turn/amplitude analysis) may also be a valuable tool for selection of target muscles, determining benefits of single and subsequent BoNT applications in the treatment of spasticity [120].

In CP children, several studies reported some benefits from BoNT injections after ES localization of appropriate muscles [121, 122]. ES is easy to perform, does not require formal EMG training, and does not prolong the procedure significantly [105]. Although the passive [123] as well as the active EMG-guided techniques have shown to be more accurate in needle placement than the manual technique, they are of limited use in children because the procedure is painful [124] and time-consuming, and requires the cooperation of the patient. Thus, it does require the patient to have sedation or mask anaesthesia. However, these techniques are used in needle placement, but it remains uncertain whether the effort to improve the BoNT injection accuracy would lead to a better response to the toxin [105].

In general, it seems that the importance of EMG or ES for guiding BoNT injections in limb muscles to treat dystonia or spasticity appeared to be based more on theoretical and preclinical data than on controlled clinical trials. Questions remain about the preferred administration of BoNT for these conditions. Future clinical researches are necessary to demonstrate a clear functional benefit of any particular injection localization method [125].

3.3. Ultrasound-guided BoNT injections

As BoNT/A is a first-line treatment for post-stroke focal spasticity, and the accuracy in delivering the toxin to the target muscles may influence the treatment outcome, a randomized clinical trial compared the reduction of upper limb spasticity using US guidance and manual needle placement (two groups of 15 stroke patients each). After one month of follow-up, the scores of the modified Ashworth scale and the finger position at rest were significantly improved in both treatment groups, although these clinical outcomes were significantly better in patients treated under US guidance [126]. In the above-mentioned randomized controlled study, manual needle placement was compared to ES- and US-guided BoNT injections into spastic forearm muscles and both US- and ES-guided techniques revealed better results than manual needle placement, but no difference was found between the two instrumental guided groups [111]. Henzel et al. (2010) compared US localization with surface landmark localization of BoNT injection in the forearm muscles in 18 spasticity patients and significant differences were observed between surface and ultrasound proximodistal and lateral coordinates for several flexor muscles, assuming that ultrasound can improve accuracy of toxin placement [113]. Another controlled trial (described more detailed above) compared manual needle placement versus ES and US guidance, but this time for the gastrocnemius muscle with better results obtained in the US group than in the ES and manual needle placement groups [112]. Ding et al. (2015) very recently explored the effectiveness of colour Doppler US-guided BoNT/A injection combined with an ankle foot brace for treating lower limb spasticity after a stroke. They found that the colour Doppler US-guided BoNT/A injection could be a safe and precise technique and a useful adjunct to the ankle foot brace treatment method [127]. US feasibility is intermediate in superficial leg muscles. It is high in forearm muscles, intrinsic hand muscles, and deep leg muscles, unless spasticity is massive and functionality is not an issue [50].

As the US-guided BoNT injection technique is easy, quick and painless, many authors suggested it might be a suitable method for use in children [105]. Moreover, according to the European consensus statement, children with CP should generally receive BoNT injections using EMG guidance or US guidance [128]. Kown et al. (2010) recently compared the clinical outcomes of ES- and US-guided localization techniques for BoNT/A gastrocnemius injections for the treatment of spastic equinus in CP children. Subscales of the physician's rating scale significantly improved in the US-guided group, but no statistical differences were noted in the modified Ashworth scale, the modified Tardieu scale, and the selective motor control. According to the authors, visual feedback by US could improve the accuracy of selective neuromuscular blocking of the gastrocnemius [129]. Besides, this guidance is preferable in children due to a better tolerability [50]. Another study compared manual needle placement with US-guided technique for BoNT injections into affected lower extremities in CP children. For the lower limb spasticity, the deep-located tibialis posterior muscle, although potentially difficult to inject, needle insertion is often performed using anatomic landmarks for guidance. Accordingly, the US anatomy of the lower leg was investigated in 25 subjects. B-mode, real-time US was performed using a 5 – 12 MHz linear array transducer. During anterior and posterior approaches, safety window width and depth were measured at the upper third and at the midpoint of the tibia. Considering the safety window width, this study suggested needle placement at the upper third of the tibia for the anterior approach and at the midpoint for the posterior approach to be safe and useful in BoNT injections [130].

US guidance of BoNT injections, however, was not solely used for limp spasticity. Chen et al. (2010) aimed to evaluate the effects of a single transrectal US-guided transperineal injection of BoNT/A to the external urethral sphincter for treating detrusor external sphincter dyssynergia in 18 patients with suprasacral spinal cord injury. There were significant reductions in integrated EMG and static and dynamic urethral pressure, but not in detrusor pressure and detrusor leak-point pressure after treatment. Postvoiding residuals also significantly decreased in the first and second month after treatment. The technique had beneficial effects in treating detrusor external sphincter dyssynergia [131]. Later on another study compared the results of a transrectal US-guided BoNT injection (18 cases) with those of a cystoscopy-guided method (20 cases) to the external urethral sphincter. Although there were no significant differences between the groups in all of the outcome measures, the study demonstrated that transrectal US-guided transperineal BoNT injection may be an alternative to a cystoscopy-guided injection. This alternative procedure provided clinicians with an innovative and less invasive method that is performed without requiring anaesthesia or cystoscopy [132]. In a non-controlled clinical trial on 19 men with sphincter hypertonia due to spinal cord injury, BoNT was injected through the transperineal way in the external urethral sphincter under EMG and transrectal US guidance, and that appeared to be an effective and safe therapeutic option [133].

It appears that although at present it is not possible to identify a golden standard among injection techniques, US guidance may be very useful in precise targeting of injections, and may help to avoid BoNT application into fat, fibrosis, vascular, and nerve structures, minimizing the spread of the toxin outside the targeted muscle belly, thus improving clinical outcomes [126]. As it is a non-invasive method, providing a relatively quick and painless muscle selection, the US-guided BoNT injection has been recommended as a standard procedure in treatment of lower leg spasticity in children with CP [50].

3.4. Endoscopy control (esophagoscopy and electromyographic guidance)

Since dysphagia and deglutition problems combined with aspiration are often caused by spasticity, hypertonus, or delayed relaxation of the upper esophageal sphincter, Schneider et al. (1994) replaced the conventional treatment including lateral cricopharyngotomy by localized BoNT injections into the cricopharyngeal muscle in a series of seven patients. For precise localization, injections were performed under general anaesthesia after location of the cricopharyngeal muscle by direct esophagoscopy and EMG guidance. Injections were administered into the dorsomedial part and on both sides into the ventrolateral parts of the muscle. All but two patients experienced complete relief or marked improvement of their complaints. There were no severe side effects or postoperative complications. This method seemed to be an effective alternative treatment to invasive procedures for patients with isolated dysfunction of the upper esophageal sphincter, and also for patients with more complex deglutition problems combined with aspiration [134].

3.5. Magnetic resonance imaging/computer tomography/fluoroscopy

MRI-, CT-, and fluoroscopy-guided procedures are typically performed by interventional radiologists [101, 135]. Because most clinicians who perform BoNT injections are not typically radiologists, US guidance of the injection is the imaging localization method routinely used. Moreover, it has several advantages in comparison with the other imaging methods, including lack of radiation, low cost, and higher accessibility, whilst providing comparable results with the mentioned imaging guiding techniques [50, 74].

4. Summary

All the studies reviewed in this chapter were quite heterogeneous regarding the characteristics of subjects and dosage, study methodology, clinical outcome measurements, and these differences hinder the possibility of performing an exact comparison or statistical analysis. Most of the studies either exploring an injection localization technique or comparing different guiding methods enrolled a small number of patients that did not allow a general unflinching recommendation to be made. The heterogeneity of muscles affected by dystonia or spasticity also contributes to the latter. However, there were some randomized, controlled clinical trials presented, but the most frequent conclusion was that there is still need of more studies in the field, so that a solid proof of the superiority of a certain localization method for BoNT injection in each specific condition can be offered.

There is informal agreement on the practicalities of BoNT injections for dystonia. The clinical examination is the simplest and most commonly applied method for localization of an overactive muscle. Based predominantly on palpation and surface anatomy, the clinical examination is usually sufficient to target a superficial muscle when not lying in close proximity to antagonistic muscles, such as most facial and some cervical muscles. Thus, it is routinely applied in the treatment of blepharospasm, some types of CD, and in many JCDs [4, 26, 106]. In these regions, EMG and imaging-guided targeting provide a second-line approach whenever refinement of muscle selection is needed or when treating a complex form [4, 71].

Although it might be beneficial, EMG is not necessary for large, superficial, easily visible muscles but is advisable for smaller and deep muscles, not readily accessible to palpation [18]. This would be the case of SD and JOD [26]. In the case of some task-specific dystonias, EMG guidance is believed to provide optimal treatment results [14]. Barbano (2001) pointed that the main advantage of needle EMG guidance is precision of toxin placement, which allows a lower dose to produce an equivalent effect. Furthermore, lower toxin doses will decrease the chance of developing neutralizing antibodies and may also allow the injection of more muscles in patients with more widespread disease [75]. However, passive EMG guidance requires selective activation of the target muscle, which is difficult to perform for patients with higher degree disturbances. In patients with dystonia and sometimes also in patients with spasticity, the co-activation of adjacent muscles may superimpose the target muscle activity. EMG guidance may be improved by ES via the injection electrode [50]. ES is the technique of choice when attempting to precisely target small muscles sited adjacent to muscles for which no BoNT effect is desired, as it is in the forearm and foot muscles. Passive EMG guidance is preferably used when injecting patients with CD or SD [12]. The disadvantages of EMG guidance include increased discomfort due to larger size of EMG needles and the lack of identification of critical structures, such as nerves and vessels and the lack of control of the applied BoNT [50]. Moreover, needle EMG is relatively invasive and may cause complications, such as bleeding and infection, and presents electrical hazards [87]. Jankovic (2001) pointed that if there is an obvious benefit of non-guided EMG BoNT treatment, a small additional improvement does not justify the routine use of EMG [14]. It is presumed that quantitative EMG-guided injections of BoNT for OMD and CD may provide treatment benefits, but very few studies, exploring the methodology, are available [46, 73]. Surface recording electrodes have been used in some trials but their recordings are limited to superficial muscles. Fine-wire electrodes have also been used, mainly for simultaneous recordings of several muscles. All these techniques are more appropriate in the research setting [26].

Recently imaging-guided BoNT injections become more popular and practiced. B-mode US allows immediate and high-resolution imaging of the injection needle position within the target region. Visual identification of muscles and depth control of needle placement are the key features of US-guided injection that lead to improved targeting and safety of BoNT applications [50, 74]. Some physicians also used the color Doppler technique in addition to the real-time B-mode scanning in order to visualize more accurate adjacent blood vessels. An emerging application is the US-guided BoNT injection into deep cervical and nuchal muscles in patients with CD, such as the scalene muscles, the longissimus cervicis muscle, and the obliquus capitis inferior muscle [50]. The use of US for locating both superficial and deep muscles is growing, as it is safe, non-invasive, and less distressing than EMG. US guidance is extremely useful when injecting muscles, adjacent to large blood vessels, or nerves, as is the case with deep cervical, forearm, and leg muscles injections [18]. The method, however, is not feasible for the pterygoid muscle and hardly feasible for the most mimic, pharyngeal, and laryngeal muscles.

Other imaging techniques, including CT or PET/CT, MRI, and fluoroscopy, are used to help accurate selection when affected muscles are deeply located (as with CD); however, these techniques are of limited value due to high costs, radiation exposure, or non-availability in daily clinical routine [71, 74].

Endoscopy-controlled BoNT injections in the terms of fiberscopy or laryngoscopy, for the treatment of SD, or as esophagoscopy in spasticity, may lead to a satisfactory treatment outcome, but often require a multidisciplinary approach that limits to some extend its use in the clinical practice [62].

Manual needle placement is still often applied in the BoNT treatment of limb spasticity. It might be sufficient in some instances when targeting large and easily accessible muscles [107], although contradictory data exist, suggesting poor success rate [114]. Thus, most studies in this area deal with electrophysiological or US techniques to optimize muscle localization for injection. Another common approach is to perform ES or EMG targeting. Similarly to focal limb dystonia, EMG is advisable for smaller and deep muscles, and it is particularly applicable in forearm and lower leg muscles and hip flexors (psoas major) [18]. Due to the listed advantages, US is considered as a valuable adjunct for muscle localization in patients with spasticity and could improve the accuracy of BoNT placement, as well. Moreover, US is already widely applied in neuropaediatric care for CP patients, as it was associated with less pain [74].

The preference of a specific localization BoNT injection method also depends on the clinical expertise of the performer, the profound knowledge on anatomy and clinical landmarks, as well as the experience in the field of EMG, US, or other more specialized disciplines as radiology and laryngology. Besides, the guiding injection technique used is not so much important in some instances as is the expertise of the physician in the field. In clinical practice, the injection guidance usage also depends on the facilities and trained personal available, as well as on the expenses incurred.

Author details

Nikolina Ilkova Semerdjieva

Address all correspondence to: nikolina.semerdjieva@gmail.com

University Hospital "St. Naum", Sofia, Bulgaria

References

[1] Simpson LL. The origin, structure, and pharmacological activity of botulinum toxin. Pharmacol Rev. 1981;33(3):155–88

[2] Jankovic J. Botulinum toxin in clinical practice. J Neurol Neurosurg Psychiatry. 2004;75(7):951–7

[3] Aoki KR, Guyer B. Botulinum toxin type A and other botulinum toxin serotypes: a comparative review of biochemical and pharmacological actions. Eur J Neurol. 2001;8(Suppl 5):21–9

[4] Guidubaldi A, Bentivoglio AR, Albanese A. Clinical use of botulinum neurotoxin: neuromuscular disorders. In: Foster KA, editor. Clinical Applications of Botulinum Neurotoxin. New York: Springer; 2014. p. 51–94

[5] Wan XH, Vuong KD, Jankovic J. Clinical application of botulinum toxin type B in movement disorders and autonomic symptoms. Chin Med Sci J. 2005;20(1):44–7

[6] Dauer WT, Burke RE, Greene P, Fahn S. Current concepts on the clinical features, aetiology and management of idiopathic cervical dystonia. Brain. 1998;121(Pt 4):547–60

[7] Warner T, Bressman S, editors. Clinical diagnosis and management of dystonia. London; Boca Raton, FL: Informa Healthcare; Distributed in North and South America by Taylor & Francis; 2007.

[8] Lapatki BG, van Dijk JP, van de Warrenburg BP, Zwarts MJ. Botulinum toxin has an increased effect when targeted toward the muscle's endplate zone: a high-density surface EMG guided study. Clin. Neurophysiol. 2011;122(8):1611–6. DOI: 10.1016/j.clinph.2010.11.018

[9] Amirali A, Mu L, Gracies JM, Simpson DM. Anatomical localization of motor endplate bands in the human biceps brachii. J Clin Neuromuscul Dis. 2007;9(2):306–12. DOI: 10.1097/CND.0b013e31815c13a7

[10] Van Campenhout A, Molenaers G. Localization of the motor endplate zone in human skeletal muscles of the lower limb: anatomical guidelines for injection with botulinum toxin. Dev Med Child Neurol. 2011;53(2):108–19. DOI: 10.1111/j.1469-8749.2010.03816.x

[11] Ye JF, Lee JH, An XC, Lin CH, Yue B, Han SH. Anatomic localization of motor entry points and accurate regions for botulinum toxin injection in the flexor digitorum superficialis. Surg Radiol Anat. 2011;33(7):601–7. DOI: 10.1007/s00276-011-0779-9

[12] Lim EC, Seet RC. Botulinum toxin: description of injection techniques and examination of controversies surrounding toxin diffusion. Acta Neurol Scand. 2008;117(2):73–84. DOI: 10.1111/j.1600-0404.2007.00931.x

[13] Jankovic J, Albanese A, Atassi MZ, Dolly JO, Hallett M, Mayer NH. Preface. Botulinum Toxin. Philadelphia: W.B. Saunders; 2009. pp. ix–x. DOI: http://dx.doi.org/10.1016/B978-1-4160-4928-9.00041-X

[14] Jankovic J. Needle EMG guidance is rarely required. Muscle & Nerve. 2001;24(11):1568–70. DOI: 10.1002/mus.1186

[15] Berardelli A, Rothwell JC, Hallett M, Thompson PD, Manfredi M, Marsden CD. The pathophysiology of primary dystonia. Brain. 1998;121(Pt 7):1195–212

[16] Tarsy D, Simon DK. Dystonia. N Engl J Med. 2006;355(8):818–29. DOI: 10.1056/NEJMra055549

[17] Simpson DM, Blitzer A, Brashear A, Comella C, Dubinsky R, Hallett M, et al. Assessment: botulinum neurotoxin for the treatment of movement disorders (an evidence-

based review): report of the Therapeutics and Technology Assessment Subcommittee of the American Academy of Neurology. Neurology. 2008;70(19):1699–706. DOI: 10.1212/01.wnl.0000311389.26145.95

[18] Ney JP, Joseph KR. Neurologic uses of botulinum neurotoxin type A. Neuropsychiatr Dis Treat. 2007;3(6):785–98

[19] Jost WH, Kohl A. Botulinum toxin: evidence-based medicine criteria in blepharospasm and hemifacial spasm. J Neurol. 2001;248(Suppl 1):21–4

[20] Ababneh OH, Cetinkaya A, Kulwin DR. Long-term efficacy and safety of botulinum toxin A injections to treat blepharospasm and hemifacial spasm. Clin Experiment Ophthalmol. 2014;42(3):254–61. DOI: 10.1111/ceo.12165

[21] Costa J, Espirito-Santo C, Borges A, Ferreira JJ, Coelho M, Moore P, et al. Botulinum toxin type A therapy for blepharospasm. Cochrane Database Syst Rev. 2005(1):CD004900. DOI: 10.1002/14651858.CD004900.pub2

[22] Balash Y, Giladi N. Efficacy of pharmacological treatment of dystonia: evidence-based review including meta-analysis of the effect of botulinum toxin and other cure options. Eur J Neurol. 2004;11(6):361–70. DOI: 10.1111/j.1468-1331.2004.00845.x

[23] Rollnik JD, Matzke M, Wohlfarth K, Dengler R, Bigalke H. Low-dose treatment of cervical dystonia, blepharospasm and facial hemispasm with albumin-diluted botulinum toxin type A under EMG guidance. An open label study. Eur Neurol. 2000;43(1): 9–12. DOI: 8121

[24] Hallett M, Albanese A, Dressler D, Segal KR, Simpson DM, Truong D, et al. Evidence-based review and assessment of botulinum neurotoxin for the treatment of movement disorders. Toxicon. 2013;67:94–114. DOI: 10.1016/j.toxicon.2012.12.004

[25] Dashtipour K, Chen JJ, Frei K, Nahab F, Tagliati M. Systematic literature review of abobotulinumtoxinA in clinical trials for blepharospasm and hemifacial spasm. Tremor Other Hyperkinet Mov (N Y). 2015;5:338. DOI: 10.7916/D8CJ8CVR

[26] Barbano RL. Anatomic Principles for Botulinum Toxin Injection. In: Stacy MA, editor. Handbook of dystonia. New York: Informa Healthcare; 2007. p. 317-40

[27] Vogt T, Lussi F, Paul A, Urban P. [Long-term therapy of focal dystonia and facial hemispasm with botulinum toxin A]. Nervenarzt. 2008;79(8):912–7. DOI: 10.1007/s00115-008-2486-2

[28] Aramideh M, Ongerboer de Visser BW, Brans JW, Koelman JH, Speelman JD. Pretarsal application of botulinum toxin for treatment of blepharospasm. J Neurol Neurosurg Psychiatry. 1995;59(3):309–11

[29] Bogucki A. [Botulinum toxin injections under electromyographic guidance]. Neurol Neurochir Pol. 1998;32(Suppl 1):85–93

[30] Blitzer A, Benson BE, Guss J, editors. Botulinum neurotoxin for head and neck disorders. New York: Thieme; 2012.

[31] Van den Bergh P, Francart J, Mourin S, Kollmann P, Laterre EC. Five-year experience in the treatment of focal movement disorders with low-dose Dysport botulinum toxin. Muscle Nerve. 1995;18(7):720–9. DOI: 10.1002/mus.880180708

[32] Sojer M, Wissel J, Muller J, Poewe W. [Treatment of focal dystonia with botulinum toxin A]. Wien Klin Wochenschr. 2001;113(Suppl 4):6–10

[33] Bhidayasiri R, Cardoso F, Truong DD. Botulinum toxin in blepharospasm and oromandibular dystonia: comparing different botulinum toxin preparations. Eur J Neurol. 2006;13(Suppl 1):21–9. DOI: 10.1111/j.1468-1331.2006.01441.x

[34] Price J, Farish S, Taylor H, O'Day J. Blepharospasm and hemifacial spasm. Randomized trial to determine the most appropriate location for botulinum toxin injections. Ophthalmology. 1997;104(5):865–8

[35] Anwar MS, Zafar H. Efficacy of botulinum toxin in benign essential blepharospasm: desirable & undesirable effects. Pak J Med Sci. 2013;29(6):1389–93

[36] Albanese A, Bentivoglio AR, Colosimo C, Galardi G, Maderna L, Tonali P. Pretarsal injections of botulinum toxin improve blepharospasm in previously unresponsive patients. J Neurol Neurosurg Psychiatry. 1996;60(6):693–4

[37] Jankovic J. Apraxia of lid opening. Mov Disord. 1995;10(5):686–7

[38] Cakmur R, Ozturk V, Uzunel F, Donmez B, Idiman F. Comparison of preseptal and pretarsal injections of botulinum toxin in the treatment of blepharospasm and hemifacial spasm. J Neurol. 2002;249(1):64–8

[39] Mackie IA. Riolan's muscle: action and indications for botulinum toxin injection. Eye (Lond). 2000;14(Pt 3A):347–52. DOI: 10.1038/eye.2000.86

[40] Patel BC, Anderson RL. Blepharospasm and related facial movement disorders. Curr Opin Ophthalmol. 1995;6(5):86–99

[41] Valls-Sole J, Tolosa ES, Ribera G. Neurophysiological observations on the effects of botulinum toxin treatment in patients with dystonic blepharospasm. J Neurol Neurosurg Psychiatry. 1991;54(4):310–3

[42] Tintner R, Jankovic J. Botulinum toxin type A in the management of oromandibular dystonia and bruxism. In: Brin M, Hallett M, Jankovic J, editors. Scientific and Therapeutic Aspects of Botulinum Toxin. Philadelphia: Lippincott Williams & Wilkins; 2002. pp. 343–50

[43] Tan EK, Jankovic J. Botulinum toxin A in patients with oromandibular dystonia: long-term follow-up. Neurology. 1999;53(9):2102–7

[44] Brin M, Blitzer A, Herman S, Steward C. Oromandibular dystonia: treatment of 96 cases with botulinum A. In: Jankovic J, Hallett M, editors. Therapy with Botulinum Toxin. New York: Marcel Dekker; 1994. pp. 429–35

[45] Rosales RL, Ng AR, Delgado-Delos Santos MM, Fernandez FF. The Broadening application of chemodenervation in X-linked dystonia-parkinsonism (Part II): an open-label experience with botulinum toxin-A (Dysport R) injections for oromandibular, lingual, and truncal-axial dystonias. Int J Neurosci. 2011;121:44–56. DOI: 10.3109/00207454.2011.558260

[46] Erdal J, Werdelin LM, Prytz S, Fuglsang-Frederiksen A, Moller E. [Botulinum toxin treatment of patients with oromandibular dystonia]. Ugeskr Laeger. 2000;162(48): 6567–71

[47] Moller E, Bakke M, Dalager T, Werdelin LM. Oromandibular dystonia involving the lateral pterygoid muscles: four cases with different complexity. Mov Disord. 2007;22(6): 785–90. DOI: 10.1002/mds.21304

[48] Odderson IR, editors. Botulinum toxin injection guide. New York: Demos Medical Pub.; 2008.

[49] Emshoff R, Bertram S, Strobl H. Ultrasonographic cross-sectional characteristics of muscles of the head and neck. Oral Surg Oral Med Oral Pathol Oral Radiol Endod. 1999;87(1):93–106

[50] Walter U, Dressler D. Ultrasound-guided botulinum toxin injections in neurology: technique, indications and future perspectives. Expert Rev Neurother. 2014;14(8):923–36. DOI: 10.1586/14737175.2014.936387

[51] Song JH, Cho ES, Kim ST, Ahn HJ. Change of distribution and timing of bite force after botulinum toxin type A injection evaluated by a computerized occlusion analysis system. Yonsei Med J. 2014;55(4):1123–9. DOI: 10.3349/ymj.2014.55.4.1123

[52] Klap P, Marion MH, Perrin A, Fresnel-Elbaz E. [Treatment of spasmodic dysphonia with botulinum toxin]. Ann Otolaryngol Chir Cervicofac. 1991;108(8):477–82; discussion 82–3

[53] Fulmer SL, Merati AL, Blumin JH. Efficacy of laryngeal botulinum toxin injection: comparison of two techniques. Laryngoscope. 2011;121(9):1924–8. DOI: 10.1002/lary.21966

[54] Srirompotong S, Saeseow P, Taweesaengsuksakul R, Kharmwan S, Srirompotong S. Botulinum toxin injection for treatment of spasmodic dysphonia: experience at Srinagarind Hospital. J Med Assoc Thai. 2006;89(12):2077–80

[55] Blitzer A. Botulinum toxin A and B: a comparative dosing study for spasmodic dysphonia. Otolaryngol Head Neck Surg. 2005;133(6):836–8. DOI: 10.1016/j.otohns.2005.09.008

[56] Morzaria S, Damrose EJ. A comparison of the VHI, VHI-10, and V-RQOL for measuring the effect of botox therapy in adductor spasmodic dysphonia. J Voice. 2012;26(3):378–80. DOI: 10.1016/j.jvoice.2010.07.011

[57] Rosow DE, Parikh P, Vivero RJ, Casiano RR, Lundy DS. Considerations for initial dosing of botulinum toxin in treatment of adductor spasmodic dysphonia. Otolaryngol Head Neck Surg. 2013;148(6):1003–6. DOI: 10.1177/0194599813484685

[58] Sulica L. Contemporary management of spasmodic dysphonia. Curr Opin Otolaryngol Head Neck Surg. 2004;12(6):543–8

[59] Hillel AD, Maronian NC, Waugh PF, Robinson L, Klotz DA. Treatment of the interarytenoid muscle with botulinum toxin for laryngeal dystonia. Ann Otol Rhinol Laryngol. 2004;113(5):341–8

[60] Meleca RJ, Hogikyan ND, Bastian RW. A comparison of methods of botulinum toxin injection for abductory spasmodic dysphonia. Otolaryngol Head Neck Surg. 1997;117(5):487–92

[61] Inagi K, Ford CN, Bless DM, Heisey D. Analysis of factors affecting botulinum toxin results in spasmodic dysphonia. J Voice. 1996;10(3):306–13

[62] Kim JW, Park JH, Park KN, Lee SW. Treatment efficacy of electromyography versus fiberscopy-guided botulinum toxin injection in adductor spasmodic dysphonia patients: a prospective comparative study. ScientificWorldJournal. 2014;2014:327928. DOI: 10.1155/2014/327928

[63] Morzaria S, Damrose EJ. The point-touch technique for botulinum toxin injection in adductor spasmodic dysphonia: quality of life assessment. J Laryngol Otol. 2011;125(7): 714–8. DOI: 10.1017/S0022215111000739

[64] Green DC, Berke GS, Ward PH, Gerratt BR. Point-touch technique of botulinum toxin injection for the treatment of spasmodic dysphonia. Ann Otol Rhinol Laryngol. 1992;101(11):883–7

[65] Sataloff RT, Mandel S, Mann EA, Ludlow CL. Practice parameter: laryngeal electromyography (an evidence-based review). Otolaryngol Head Neck Surg. 2004;130(6): 770–9. DOI: 10.1016/j.otohns.2004.04.003

[66] Zielinska M, Selmaj K. [A case of laryngeal adductor dystonia treated with transcutaneous injections of botulinum toxin]. Neurol Neurochir Pol. 1998;32(5):1273–80

[67] Blitzer A, Brin MF, Stewart C, Aviv JE, Fahn S. Abductor laryngeal dystonia: a series treated with botulinum toxin. Laryngoscope. 1992;102(2):163–7. DOI: 10.1288/00005537-199202000-00011

[68] Bielamowicz S, Squire S, Bidus K, Ludlow CL. Assessment of posterior cricoarytenoid botulinum toxin injections in patients with abductor spasmodic dysphonia. Ann Otol Rhinol Laryngol. 2001;110(5 Pt 1):406–12

[69] Persaud R, Garas G, Silva S, Stamatoglou C, Chatrath P, Patel K. An evidence-based review of botulinum toxin (Botox) applications in non-cosmetic head and neck conditions. JRSM Short Rep. 2013;4(2):10. DOI: 10.1177/2042533312472115

[70] Galardi G, Guerriero R, Amadio S, Leocani L, Teggi R, Melloni G, et al. Sporadic failure of botulinum toxin treatment in usually responsive patients with adductor spasmodic dysphonia. Neurol Sci. 2001;22(4):303–6

[71] Lee IH, Yoon YC, Sung DH, Kwon JW, Jung JY. Initial experience with imaging-guided intramuscular botulinum toxin injection in patients with idiopathic cervical dystonia. AJR Am J Roentgenol. 2009;192(4):996–1001. DOI: 10.2214/AJR.08.1535

[72] Mezaki T. [Clinical application of botulinum toxin]. Brain Nerve. 2011;63(7):785–94

[73] Nijmeijer SW, Koelman JH, Kamphuis DJ, Tijssen MA. Muscle selection for treatment of cervical dystonia with botulinum toxin--a systematic review. Parkinsonism Relat Disord. 2012;18(6):731–6. DOI: 10.1016/j.parkreldis.2012.04.005

[74] Schramm A, Baumer T, Fietzek U, Heitmann S, Walter U, Jost WH. Relevance of sonography for botulinum toxin treatment of cervical dystonia: an expert statement. J Neural Transm (Vienna). 2015;122(10):1457–63. DOI: 10.1007/s00702-014-1356-2

[75] Barbano RL. Needle EMG guidance for injection of botulinum toxin. Needle EMG guidance is useful. Muscle Nerve. 2001;24(11):1567–8

[76] Speelman JD, Brans JW. Cervical dystonia and botulinum treatment: is electromyographic guidance necessary? Mov Disord. 1995;10(6):802. DOI: 10.1002/mds.870100619

[77] Wulff CH, Dupont E. [Torticollis treated with botulinum toxin]. Ugeskr Laeger. 1993;155(5):284–9

[78] Dubinsky RM, Gray CS, Vetere-Overfield B, Koller WC. Electromyographic guidance of botulinum toxin treatment in cervical dystonia. Clin Neuropharmacol. 1991;14(3): 262–7

[79] Comella CL, Buchman AS, Tanner CM, Brown-Toms NC, Goetz CG. Botulinum toxin injection for spasmodic torticollis: increased magnitude of benefit with electromyographic assistance. Neurology. 1992;42(4):878–82

[80] Lee LH, Chang WN, Chang CS. The finding and evaluation of EMG-guided BOTOX injection in cervical dystonia. Acta Neurol Taiwan. 2004;13(2):71–6

[81] Werdelin L, Dalager T, Fuglsang-Frederiksen A, Regeur L, Karlsborg M, Korbo L, et al. The utility of EMG interference pattern analysis in botulinum toxin treatment of torticollis: a randomised, controlled and blinded study. Clin Neurophysiol. 2011;122(11):2305–9. DOI: 10.1016/j.clinph.2011.04.012

[82] Cordivari C, Misra VP, Vincent A, Catania S, Bhatia KP, Lees AJ. Secondary nonresponsiveness to botulinum toxin A in cervical dystonia: the role of electromyogram-

guided injections, botulinum toxin A antibody assay, and the extensor digitorum brevis test. Mov Disord. 2006;21(10):1737–41. DOI: 10.1002/mds.21051

[83] Mezaki T, Matsumoto S, Sakamoto T, Mizutani K, Kaji R. [Cervical echomyography in cervical dystonia and its application to the monitoring for muscle afferent block (MAB)]. Rinsho Shinkeigaku. 2000;40(7):689–93

[84] Hong JS, Sathe GG, Niyonkuru C, Munin MC. Elimination of dysphagia using ultrasound guidance for botulinum toxin injections in cervical dystonia. Muscle Nerve. 2012;46(4):535–9. DOI: 10.1002/mus.23409

[85] Herting B, Wunderlich S, Glockler T, Bendszus M, Mucha D, Reichmann H, et al. Computed tomographically-controlled injection of botulinum toxin into the longus colli muscle in severe anterocollis. Mov Disord. 2004;19(5):588–90. DOI: 10.1002/mds.10704

[86] Pappas GP, Olcott EW, Drace JE. Imaging of skeletal muscle function using (18)FDG PET: force production, activation, and metabolism. J Appl Physiol (1985). 2001;90(1): 329-37

[87] Sung DH, Choi JY, Kim DH, Kim ES, Son YI, Cho YS, et al. Localization of dystonic muscles with 18F-FDG PET/CT in idiopathic cervical dystonia. J Nucl Med. 2007;48(11): 1790–5. DOI: 10.2967/jnumed.107.044024

[88] Glass GA, Ku S, Ostrem JL, Heath S, Larson PS. Fluoroscopic, EMG-guided injection of botulinum toxin into the longus colli for the treatment of anterocollis. Parkinsonism Relat Disord. 2009;15(8):610–3. DOI: 10.1016/j.parkreldis.2009.01.006

[89] Karp BI. Botulinum toxin treatment of occupational and focal hand dystonia. Mov Disord. 2004;19(Suppl 8):S116–9. DOI: 10.1002/mds.20025

[90] Kruisdijk JJ, Koelman JH, Ongerboer de Visser BW, de Haan RJ, Speelman JD. Botulinum toxin for writer's cramp: a randomised, placebo-controlled trial and 1-year follow-up. J Neurol Neurosurg Psychiatry. 2007;78(3):264–70. DOI: 10.1136/jnnp.2005.083170

[91] Sherman AL, Willick SP, Cardenas DD. Management of focal dystonia of the extensor hallucis longus muscle with botulinum toxin injection: a case report. Arch Phys Med Rehabil. 1998;79(10):1303–5

[92] Chen R, Karp BI, Hallett M. Botulinum toxin type F for treatment of dystonia: long-term experience. Neurology. 1998;51(5):1494-6

[93] Yoshimura DM, Aminoff MJ, Olney RK. Botulinum toxin therapy for limb dystonias. Neurology. 1992;42(3 Pt 1):627–30

[94] Tsui JK, Bhatt M, Calne S, Calne DB. Botulinum toxin in the treatment of writer's cramp: a double-blind study. Neurology. 1993;43(1):183–5

[95] Molloy FM, Shill HA, Kaelin-Lang A, Karp BI. Accuracy of muscle localization without EMG: implications for treatment of limb dystonia. Neurology. 2002;58(5):805–7

[96] Schuele S, Jabusch HC, Lederman RJ, Altenmuller E. Botulinum toxin injections in the treatment of musician's dystonia. Neurology. 2005;64(2):341–3. DOI: 10.1212/01.WNL.0000149768.36634.92

[97] Geenen C, Consky E, Ashby P. Localizing muscles for botulinum toxin treatment of focal hand dystonia. Can J Neurol Sci. 1996;23(3):194–7

[98] Cohen LG, Hallett M, Geller BD, Hochberg F. Treatment of focal dystonias of the hand with botulinum toxin injections. J Neurol Neurosurg Psychiatry. 1989;52(3):355–63

[99] Ross MH, Charness ME, Sudarsky L, Logigian EL. Treatment of occupational cramp with botulinum toxin: diffusion of toxin to adjacent noninjected muscles. Muscle Nerve. 1997;20(5):593–8

[100] Lim EC, Quek AM, Seet RC. Accurate targeting of botulinum toxin injections: how to and why. Parkinsonism Relat Disord. 2011;17(Suppl 1):S34–9. DOI: 10.1016/j.parkreldis.2011.06.016

[101] Mokhtari S, Hugeron C, Roffi F, Thibaut JB, Le Breton C, Mompoint D, et al. [Spasticity: clinical and imaging features]. J Radiol. 2010;91(12 Pt 2):1387–97

[102] Walker HW, Lee MY, Bahroo LB, Hedera P, Charles D. Botulinum toxin injection techniques for the management of adult spasticity. PM R. 2015;7(4):417–27. DOI: 10.1016/j.pmrj.2014.09.021

[103] Muller F, Cugy E, Ducerf C, Delleci C, Guehl D, Joseph PA, et al. Safety and self-reported efficacy of botulinum toxin for adult spasticity in current clinical practice: a prospective observational study. Clin Rehabil. 2012;26(2):174–9. DOI: 10.1177/0269215511412799

[104] Warnink-Kavelaars J, Vermeulen RJ, Becher JG. Study protocol: precision of a protocol for manual intramuscular needle placement checked by passive stretching and relaxing of the target muscle in the lower extremity during BTX-A treatment in children with spastic cerebral palsy, as verified by means of electrical stimulation. BMC Pediatr. 2013;13:129. DOI: 10.1186/1471-2431-13-129

[105] Park ES, Rha DW. Botulinum toxin type A injection for management of upper limb spasticity in children with cerebral palsy: a literature review. Yonsei Med J. 2006;47(5):589–603. DOI: 10.3349/ymj.2006.47.5.589

[106] Chin TY, Nattrass GR, Selber P, Graham HK. Accuracy of intramuscular injection of botulinum toxin A in juvenile cerebral palsy: a comparison between manual needle placement and placement guided by electrical stimulation. J Pediatr Orthop. 2005;25(3):286–91

[107] Mall V, Heinen F, Siebel A, Bertram C, Hafkemeyer U, Wissel J, et al. Treatment of adductor spasticity with BTX-A in children with CP: a randomized, double-blind, placebo-controlled study. Dev Med Child Neurol. 2006;48(1):10–3. DOI: 10.1017/S0012162206000041

[108] Yang EJ, Rha DW, Yoo JK, Park ES. Accuracy of manual needle placement for gastrocnemius muscle in children with cerebral palsy checked against ultrasonography. Arch Phys Med Rehabil. 2009;90(5):741–4. DOI: 10.1016/j.apmr.2008.10.025

[109] Kaishou X, Tiebin Y, Jianning M. A randomized controlled trial to compare two botulinum toxin injection techniques on the functional improvement of the leg of children with cerebral palsy. Clin Rehabil. 2009;23(9):800–11. DOI: 10.1177/0269215509335295

[110] Childers MK, Stacy M, Cooke DL, Stonnington HH. Comparison of two injection techniques using botulinum toxin in spastic hemiplegia. Am J Phys Med Rehabil. 1996;75(6):462–9

[111] Picelli A, Lobba D, Midiri A, Prandi P, Melotti C, Baldessarelli S, et al. Botulinum toxin injection into the forearm muscles for wrist and fingers spastic overactivity in adults with chronic stroke: a randomized controlled trial comparing three injection techniques. Clin Rehabil. 2014;28(3):232–42. DOI: 10.1177/0269215513497735

[112] Picelli A, Tamburin S, Bonetti P, Fontana C, Barausse M, Dambruoso F, et al. Botulinum toxin type A injection into the gastrocnemius muscle for spastic equinus in adults with stroke: a randomized controlled trial comparing manual needle placement, electrical stimulation and ultrasonography-guided injection techniques. Am J Phys Med Rehabil. 2012;91(11):957–64. DOI: 10.1097/PHM.0b013e318269d7f3

[113] Henzel MK, Munin MC, Niyonkuru C, Skidmore ER, Weber DJ, Zafonte RD. Comparison of surface and ultrasound localization to identify forearm flexor muscles for botulinum toxin injections. PM R. 2010;2(7):642–6. DOI: 10.1016/j.pmrj.2010.05.002

[114] Schnitzler A, Roche N, Denormandie P, Lautridou C, Parratte B, Genet F. Manual needle placement: accuracy of botulinum toxin A injections. Muscle Nerve. 2012;46(4):531–4. DOI: 10.1002/mus.23410

[115] Rodriquez AA, McGinn M, Chappell R. Botulinum toxin injection of spastic finger flexors in hemiplegic patients. Am J Phys Med Rehabil. 2000;79(1):44–7

[116] Palmer DT, Horn LJ, Harmon RL. Botulinum toxin treatment of lumbrical spasticity: a brief report. Am J Phys Med Rehabil. 1998;77(4):348–50

[117] Richardson D, Edwards S, Sheean GL, Greenwood RJ, Thompson AJ. The effect of botulinum toxin on hand function after incomplete spinal cord injury at the level of C5/6: a case report. Clin Rehabil. 1997;11(4):288–92

[118] Hesse S, Lucke D, Malezic M, Bertelt C, Friedrich H, Gregoric M, et al. Botulinum toxin treatment for lower limb extensor spasticity in chronic hemiparetic patients. J Neurol Neurosurg Psychiatry. 1994;57(11):1321–4

[119] Dunne JW, Heye N, Dunne SL. Treatment of chronic limb spasticity with botulinum toxin A. J Neurol Neurosurg Psychiatry. 1995;58(2):232–5

[120] Finsterer J, Fuchs I, Mamoli B. Automatic EMG-guided botulinum toxin treatment of spasticity. Clin Neuropharmacol. 1997;20(3):195–203

[121] Wallen MA, O'Flaherty S J, Waugh MC. Functional outcomes of intramuscular botulinum toxin type A in the upper limbs of children with cerebral palsy: a phase II trial. Arch Phys Med Rehabil. 2004;85(2):192–200

[122] Speth LA, Leffers P, Janssen-Potten YJ, Vles JS. Botulinum toxin A and upper limb functional skills in hemiparetic cerebral palsy: a randomized trial in children receiving intensive therapy. Dev Med Child Neurol. 2005;47(7):468–73

[123] Autti-Ramo I, Larsen A, Taimo A, von Wendt L. Management of the upper limb with botulinum toxin type A in children with spastic type cerebral palsy and acquired brain injury: clinical implications. Eur J Neurol. 2001;8(Suppl 5):136–44

[124] Bayon-Mottu M, Gambart G, Deries X, Tessiot C, Richard I, Dinomais M. Pain during injections of botulinum toxin in children: influence of the localization technique. Ann Phys Rehabil Med. 2014;57(9–10):578–86. DOI: 10.1016/j.rehab.2014.09.010

[125] Childers MK. The importance of electromyographic guidance and electrical stimulation for injection of botulinum toxin. Phys Med Rehabil Clin N Am. 2003;14(4):781–92

[126] Santamato A, Micello MF, Panza F, Fortunato F, Baricich A, Cisari C, et al. Can botulinum toxin type A injection technique influence the clinical outcome of patients with post-stroke upper limb spasticity? A randomized controlled trial comparing manual needle placement and ultrasound-guided injection techniques. J Neurol Sci. 2014;347(1–2):39–43. DOI: 10.1016/j.jns.2014.09.016

[127] Ding XD, Zhang GB, Chen HX, Wang W, Song JH, Fu DG. Color Doppler ultrasound-guided botulinum toxin type A injection combined with an ankle foot brace for treating lower limb spasticity after a stroke. Eur Rev Med Pharmacol Sci. 2015;19(3):406–11

[128] Heinen F, Desloovere K, Schroeder AS, Berweck S, Borggraefe I, van Campenhout A, et al. The updated European Consensus 2009 on the use of Botulinum toxin for children with cerebral palsy. Eur J Paediatr Neurol. 2010;14(1):45–66. DOI: 10.1016/j.ejpn.2009.09.005

[129] Kwon JY, Hwang JH, Kim JS. Botulinum toxin a injection into calf muscles for treatment of spastic equinus in cerebral palsy: a controlled trial comparing sonography and electric stimulation-guided injection techniques: a preliminary report. Am J Phys Med Rehabil. 2010;89(4):279–86. DOI: 10.1097/PHM.0b013e3181ca24ac

[130] Rha DW, Park ES, Jung S, Lee SC, Suh M, Choi HS. Comparison of ultrasound-guided anterior and posterior approaches for needle insertion into the tibialis posterior in hemiplegic children with spastic cerebral palsy. Am J Phys Med Rehabil. 2014;93(10): 841–8. DOI: 10.1097/PHM.0000000000000170

[131] Chen SL, Bih LI, Chen GD, Huang YH, You YH, Lew HL. Transrectal ultrasound-guided transperineal botulinum toxin a injection to the external urethral sphincter for treat-

ment of detrusor external sphincter dyssynergia in patients with spinal cord injury. Arch Phys Med Rehabil. 2010;91(3):340–4. DOI: 10.1016/j.apmr.2009.11.006

[132] Chen SL, Bih LI, Chen GD, Huang YH, You YH. Comparing a transrectal ultrasound-guided with a cystoscopy-guided botulinum toxin a injection in treating detrusor external sphincter dyssynergia in spinal cord injury. Am J Phys Med Rehabil. 2011;90(9): 723–30. DOI: 10.1097/PHM.0b013e31821a72a3

[133] Romero-Culleres G, Conejero-Sugranes J, Gonzalez-Viejo MA, Bruno-Montoro J, Lopez-Guillen P, Abenoza-Guardiola M. [Efficacy and safety of botulinum toxin in external urethral sphincter by transperineal way guided transrectal ultrasound and electromyography on chronic urinary retention due to spinal cord injury]. Med Clin (Barc). 2011;137(8):346–8. DOI: 10.1016/j.medcli.2010.10.025

[134] Schneider I, Thumfart WF, Pototschnig C, Eckel HE. Treatment of dysfunction of the cricopharyngeal muscle with botulinum A toxin: introduction of a new, noninvasive method. Ann Otol Rhinol Laryngol. 1994;103(1):31–5

[135] Brant CQ, Siqueira ES, Ferrari AP, Jr. Botulinum toxin for oropharyngeal dysphagia: case report of flexible endoscope-guided injection. Dis Esophagus. 1999;12(1):68–73